Post-pelleting application of liquid additives

Acknowledgements

The authors would like to thank G. Eijsermans, K. Ouwerkerk, B. van der Pol, E. van Leeuwen and M.A.K. Maes for their useful practical information from the compoounf feed industry and machine builders point of view and Prof.Dr.Ir. M.W.A. Verstegen for his comments on the booklet.

Wageningen Feed Processing Centre

The Wageningen Feed Processing Centre (WFPC) represents a research collaboration between the Departments of Animal Nutrition and Process Engineering on animal feed science, technology and nutrition.

A focal point of WFPC research is the advocacy of an increasingly process-technology oriented approach towards animal feed production and research.

This approach leads to a better insight into processes and to better control and regulation. It additionally provides greater certainty about compliance with the requirements of quality assurance systems, leading to increased cost efficiency and resulting in a more reliable production planning.

The main areas of WFPC research are as follows:
- Feed production engineering
- Process (system) development
- Nutritional evaluation of processing effects

WFPC Office

Wageningen Feed Processing Centre
Marijkeweg 40
6709 PG Wageningen
The Netherlands

Phone	+31 317 484156
Fax	+31 317 484260
e-Mail	wfpc@alg.vv.wau.nl
Internet	http://www.zod.wau.nl/~www-vv/wfpc/wfpc.html

Post-pelleting application of liquid additives

of liquid additives

G.M.A. Engelen
A.F.B. van der Poel

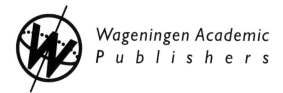

Wageningen Academic
P u b l i s h e r s

ISBN 978-90-74134-66-8

www.WageningenAcademic.com

First published, 1999
Reprint, 2007

Wageningen Academic Publishers
The Netherlands, 2007

PREFACE

This report is the result of a research project of the Animal Nutrition Group of the Department of Animal Sciences. The research has involved the technology of the addition of liquid additives on pelleted feed in post-pelleting applications.

It is the mission of the Wageningen Institute of Animal Sciences (WIAS) to contribute to the sustainability of animal production through fundamental and strategic research and education. Within its Animal Nutrition Group, the nutrition of ruminants, of pigs/poultry and animal feed technology are three key topics of research.

Fundamental and applied research on animal feed technology has been carried out since 1984 and has been expanded since facilities at the Wageningen Feed Processing Centre (WFPC) were installed in 1993 to study the nutritional, hygienic and physical quality of animal feeds, as affected by thermal and other process treatments. Since then, research efforts have been increased and the research centre has become a flexible and successful operation.

The base of animal production is the feed. The feed industry therefore has an important task to fulfil to guarantee sustainability for now and for the future. Sustainability of animal production has to be associated with cost effectiveness, environmental impact and quality. In achieving these goals, the feed of the animal has a major influence. Therefore the feed industry as the start of the food chain is obligated to improve the quality, cost effectiveness and digestibility/utilisation of animal feed, to decrease the environmental impact of waste products. With this research the authors hope to contribute to meeting these challenges in producing animal feed. With the use of feed additives the cost effectiveness and digestibility/utilisation can be improved. These feed additives, however, are often sensitive to thermal processing.

Post-pelleting addition of heat sensitive additives is a way to avoid damage to additives. It also contributes to the reduction of carry-over and cross contamination. The use of liquid additives in a post-pelleting application (PPA) may be an alternative technological solution whereby an even dosing of an additive into animal feed can be provided together with a virtual 100% recovery of the additive. This will ultimately benefit the feed manufacturer since it will provide more flexibility in terms of the demand for special custom-built feeds.

In the period from October 1997 to October 1998, Guus Engelen has worked on research involving liquid additives in post-pelleting applications at the Wageningen Feed Processing Centre. This was part of his Agricultural Engineering study. The thesis written on this research has led to this booklet with the help of Thomas van der Poel.

This booklet presents a compilation of the literature associated with the use of liquid additives in animal feed. The implementation of liquid additive systems gives rise to a number of requirements for both feed and equipment, which will be discussed in detail after a general discussion and a definition of quality. At the end a list of references is included. The booklet can be used as a ready reference by process engineers, nutritionists, researchers and students who are interested in post-pelleting applications of additives, in the production line and its design.

The authors hope that this booklet will provide a useful entry to the literature of liquid additive dosing in post-pelleting applications, as some of the more general effects and information have also been included. We hope that it may have a valuable role as a source of information and ideas for research & development and serve as a means of extending these.

Guus Engelen
Thomas van der Poel

TABLE OF CONTENTS

SUMMARY

The application of micro-ingredients and especially well defined enzymes is expanding into an important and indispensable tool for the animal feed industry. The incorporation of micro ingredients as a dry product during the mixing stage of the feed manufacturing process is in general practice. Increased treatment intensities are used in the routine manufacturing of compound feed for different reasons such as improving pellet quality and salmonella decontamination. These treatment intensities are, however, not relevant for proper inclusion of feed additives. Therefore, the addition of (heat-sensitive) additives after intensive treatment of the feed is an alternative to avoid damage to the additive, and has a role in the reduction of carry-over and cross contamination (Heidenreich, 1995).

The application of liquid additives in a post-pelleting application (PPA) may be an alternative technological solution in the case an even dosing of the additive into the feed and virtually 100% recovery of the additives used can be attained (Günther and Beudeker, 1997; Barendse, 1995; Gill, 1994). This will ultimately benefit the feed manufacturer as it will provide more flexibility towards the increasing demand for special custom-built feeds. This is definitely the case with bulk-blending, a relatively new step in the production process, where semi-finished products or raw materials are mixed, fat coated and sprayed with additives after storage of the (semi-)finished products and shortly before loading (Van der Steege, 1998).

The implementation of liquid addition systems, however, adds a number of requirements to feed and equipment. At the moment, the additives are not all available in a fluid form. According to one of the producers there is intensive research into fluid formulations, but this needs time and will not be ready in the short run (Wagner, 1998). Besides that, dosing levels in general are very low and there is very little information known about the compatibility of liquid additives in mixtures.

Harker (1995) found that an underdose as well as an overdose of enzyme has a negative effect on the cost-effective production of broilers. Accordingly, the uniformity of the enzyme-sprayed feed is very important. The coefficient of variation in feed samples from the normal day ration of the target animal should not be more than 10% (Beumer, 1991; Wicker and Poole, 1991; Barendse, 1993; Günther and Beudeker, 1997; Heidenreich, 1998).

There are possibilities for continuous as well as discontinuous post-pelleting applications. The industry, however, has to be cautious with the implementation of post-pelleting applications. The choice of dry or liquid addition of feed additive needs, is not as simple as price or convenience because they have a major impact (Blair, 1996). The quality of liquid addition has an impact on feed intake as well as on animal performance. These items in particular have to be examined in relation with different types of feed additives. It can be concluded that further investigations regarding the uniformity, contamination and separation are important to determine the field of application.

1 INTRODUCTION

1.1 THE COMPOUND FEED INDUSTRY

For the composition of compound feed for livestock, a mixture is made out of different components with a desirable content of the different energy and nutrients in conformance with feeding standards and current scientific views. The recipes of compound feeds are formulated out of the main or macro-components such as grains, soya and so on, dosed in certain percentages and not very critical in contamination (Robohm, 1998). Besides that, these mixtures contain micro-components, the so-called additives, which are added in a range of mg/kg (Von Gerlach, 1992). The macro-components are usually part of any recipe and carry-over of macro-components then only changes the contents in the batch mixture, while micro-components are desirable in many recipes, but completely intolerable in others. Therefore micro-components are very sensitive to contamination and carry-over (Robohm, 1998).

The purpose of these micro-components is to enhance animal health and animal production. Known micro-components are trace elements, vitamins and pharmaceutical compounds. The preparation of these mixtures with a very low content of micro-components requires a high level of working accuracy, to recover these components completely and to establish an even distribution (Von Gerlach, 1992).

In modern agricultural livestock production, the most important issue is cost-effectiveness. Due to small profit margins, there is a constant drive to obtain low-cost feeds with optimal nutrient availability. As a consequence, the compound feed industry has a continuous interest in processing cheap agricultural products and by-products into valuable feed ingredients. As will be shown in subsequent sections, the application of well defined feed enzymes and additives is growing into an important and indispensable tool for these feed producers (Van Dijck and Geerse, 1993).

In addition to cost-effectiveness, issues of environmental concern have become important, especially in those regions of the world with dense animal and human populations. Examples of such areas are the Netherlands, parts of Brittany in France, Northwest Germany, the Po region in Italy, and some parts of Taiwan. In the Netherlands, legislation on air, soil and ground-water pollution by animal manure has created a need for the development of cost-effective enzymes alleviating these problems; other problem areas will follow in due time (Van Dijck and Geerse, 1993). The bases of animal production must be conserved in order for animal production to be possible into the future. Sustainability cannot be equated with a low production level, extensive farming and government-controlled restriction of production, although it cannot be denied that extensive farming does in fact contain elements of sustainability. The yardstick is, however, the task to be fulfilled, for example feeding the still growing number of people on this earth (Peisker, 1998).

1.2 DEVELOPMENTS IN THE FUTURE

Flexibility in the compound feed industry is necessary to be able to cope with the specific wishes of the farmer and the demand for safe feed (Heijnen according to Van Vliet, 1998; Anonymous, 1998a). Consumers have higher demands on foodstuffs. The food-chain is more and more influenced by the primary agricultural sector. The market, therefore, forces the compound industry to (Heijnen, 1998a):
- Produce compound feed that is not contaminated;
- Achieve higher hygiene standards;
- Achieve a minimal load on the environment.

A growing percentage of farmers have mixing equipment available themselves. Especially when we look at the feed-mill-mix installations on pig farms, a considerable increase is recognised. In the seasons 1994/1995 and 1995/1996 the percentage of on-farm mixing increased from 1.6 to 4.6, and the development is still continuing (Coops, 1997). After the introduction of the MacSharry-policy in 1994, grain has become cheaper and it was attractive to replace a part of the concentrates and by-products with wheat or barley (Gengler, 1996). If we take into account that the compound feed market is decreasing, for example decreasing the number of pigs by Dutch law, an adaptation in the assortment will be necessary for the compound feed manufacturer (Coops, 1997). This will result in a growing number of types of feed, more and more small batches and order-controlled production (Robohm, 1998; Van der Steege, 1998). Also increased knowledge of animal farming and a scaling-up in animal husbandry plays an important role: it makes the profitability of the compound feed industry even more difficult (Coops, 1997).

The growing increase of the product assortment can be realised by different options (Coops, 1997):
- Produce more types of feed on the same production line;
- Produce more basic types of feed and mix these in a bulk station using certain proportions, possibly with additives;
- Co-operate with other compound feed producers.

In the first option the direct result is a drastic capacity decrease. Besides that, problems of contamination and storage increase: more small storage cells are required; and different feeds on one feed line increase the risk of carry-over. The second option requires a certain investment. Still, many problems can be solved with this option, where it is possible to achieve less contamination and higher hygiene standards. This option may require a greater loading time. The third possibility has logistical problems and is socially/emotionally very sensitive (Coops, 1997).

1.3 DESCRIPTION OF PROBLEMS ASSOCIATED WITH ADDITION OF MICRO-COMPONENTS

To satisfy hygiene requirements and good feed quality, high temperatures are used during the preparation of feed. For example because of recent public health concern notably over salmonella, some feed manufacturers are now pelleting at temperatures in excess of 90 °C (Perry, 1997); pelleting between 60 and 80 °C is currently not uncommon (Peisker, 1993). Classical pelleting involves conditioning, pressing and cooling the feed mixture, but more and more modifications to conventional pelleting techniques are being used today, such as double pressing or the application of alternative conditioning processes. Additionally the number of highly intensive short-term treatment systems, besides pelleting, for the compound feed industry is still increasing. The thermal treatment of *single* components and mixtures has a lot of advantages (Peisker, 1995; Schwarz, 1998a):
- Gelatinisation of starch;
- Hygiene treatment;
- Enhancing the pellet quality and the press capacity;
- Enhancing digestibility;
- Reducing antinutritional factors.

These additional thermal treatments are often performed in an expander (König, 1995), toaster or extruder line. These technologies combine a higher process temperature with the addition of steam and high pressure (Robohm, 1998). The intensity of processing affects for example the number of enterobacteriaceae (salmonellae) in feed (König, 1995; Heidenreich and Löwe, 1994); shown in figure 1.1. Heidenreich and Löwe (1994) concluded that in processing at temperatures from 115-125 °C decontamination of salmonellae was relatively effective.

The various stress factors, coming together with more intensive processing (See Annex A) are mainly of a hydro-thermal or mechanical nature and have a more or less severe influence on the stability of a range of additives and other micro-components. Heat, moisture, pressure and friction, reduction and oxidation reactions and light are stress factors which can negatively influence additives (Schwarz, 1998a; Putnam and Taylor, 1997; Perry, 1997; Blair, 1996; Liebert et al., 1993). Application of heat sensitive additives like enzymes, vitamins, aromates, amino acids, probiotics and antibiotics, therefore desires different process routes in the compound industry (Van der Poel, 1996).

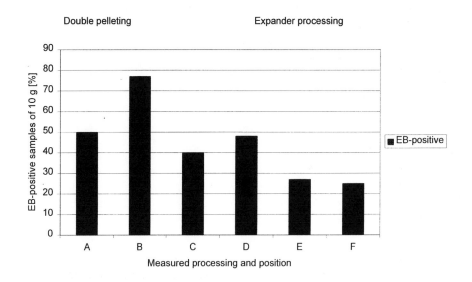

Figure 1.1 Enterobacteriaceae (EB)-positive samples in 10 g feed after double pelleting and expander processing.

A   Pellets after double pelleting, not cooled
B   Pellets after double pelleting, cooled
C   Expanded feed, not cooled
D   Expanded feed, cooled
E   pelleted expanded feed, not cooled
F   pelleted expanded feed, cooled

Reference: Heidenreich and Löwe, 1994.

At high temperatures it is useful to bring the enzymes into the feed after pelleting (Post-Pelleting-Application, in short PPA). This can also be done for the other heat sensitive additives (Barendse and Van Doesum, 1993). This approach enables the industry to avoid loss of effectiveness of the additive during pre-treatment and pelleting of the feed (Barendse, 1995). On the basis of an insufficient thermo-stability, additives cannot be added in the mash-feed via a premix without activity loss being noticed. When the feed is processed at temperatures above 75 °C, unacceptable activity losses or even a total loss may take place (Günther and Beudeker, 1997). PPA processes are therefore implemented more and more (Barendse, 1995). The application of liquid additives after pelleting may be an alternative technological solution if an even dosing of the additive into the feed and virtually 100% recovery of the added additive can be provided (Van der Poel and Engelen, 1998).

The critical factor in the post-pelleting application is the amount of additive that needs to be available in every portion of feed. Both an overdose and a shortage are undesirable. The coefficient of variation in feed samples from the day ration of the target animal should not be more than 10% (Beumer, 1991; Wicker and Poole, 1991; Barendse, 1993; Günther and Beudeker, 1997; Heidenreich, 1998).

In the compound feed industry and the machine builders there is a lack of knowledge about the effectiveness in addition of liquid additives in a PPA. On one hand, a lack in terms of design of the installation and on the other hand in terms of the effectiveness of liquid additives in comparison with powder additives that have had a heat treatment. The compound industry, and also the machine designers have a task of improving the performance of the machines, especially quality performance (Heeres and Vahl, 1997).

Post-pelleting application is not completely new for the industry: fats and flavours have been added to feed in post-pelleting applications for a number of years now. The spraying of, for example, enzymes and antibiotics requires more accuracy than the spraying of fats and flavours. Fat is sprayed on the pellets in amounts from 1 to 3% of the feed (Barendse and Van Doesum, 1993); and for fish feeds in even higher percentages (Eijsermans, 1997). Enzymes are added in amounts varying from 0.002% to 0.1% of the feed.

The success of a PPA installation fundamentally depends on two things:
- development and availability of suitable premixes in liquid form, chapter 3;
- precise functioning high standard technical equipment, chapter 4.

In order to be successful in achieving a high quality of feed as well as animal product (chapter 2), a good co-operation between these two factors is absolutely necessary (Abele, 1996).

2 QUALITY DETERMINED BY FEED

Quality control in the case of products and processes plays an increasing role in society under influence of consumer demands. Also in animal production as a part of the food chain this is becoming more and more important. Current points of attention are quality care in compound feed production, the dairy chain, meat production and animal health are. Certification in quality control is getting more and more important in these fields (Anonymous, 1997a).

2.1 QUALITY IN THE COMPOUND FEED INDUSTRY

The easiest way of controlling quality in the compound feed industry is inspection for errors in the end product or during processing. A second form of quality control is process-control, characterised by optimising the production process, controlling and analysing the raw materials and feed back of the mistakes. To have a reference window, quality standards are formulated, such as NEN/ISO 9000 to 9004. These are mostly restricted to the technical part of the industry. A third, most intensive, quality control measure is the integral quality control that takes the consumers demand as a start-point. Thinking in terms of quality means in fact thinking in terms of goals. One can define three conditions for formulating quality objectives (Van der Poel, 1997):
1. Measurability; necessary for the control of the realisation of the objectives;
2. Controllability; it is no use putting energy in uncontrollable objectives;
3. Visibility; objectives need to be visible in a short term for the persons responsible.

The formulation of the GMP-codes (Good Manufacturing Practices) in 1991/92 was the direct result of an increasing consciousness-raising in the animal feed sector as a part of the whole feed-to-food production chain (Anonymous, 1997a).

The quality system of a company is the organising and documenting of responsibilities, procedures, processes and facilities in relation to realising control and guarantee of a basic quality of compound feed. One of the requirements is making a GMP hand out that needs to contain (Van der Poel, 1997):
- Specifications of raw materials, premixes and other used products;
- Schematic representation of the process line and its critical points;
- Specifications of the compound feeds to deliver;
- Definition of all necessary inspections from raw material to end product on the critical points including storage and transport;
- Definition of the measurement techniques used for inspection.

For application of additives there is a special module in the GMP-codes that states the next objectives (Heeres and Vahl, 1997):
- Using the right additives and veterinary products;
- In the right dosage/accuracy;
- Uniformity/homogeneity;
- An acceptable level of contamination;
- Processed in the right compound feed.

Objectives 1 and 5 exceed the aim of this study but attention will be paid to objectives 2, 3 and 4.

Right dosage or accuracy
If dosing and balancing is performed automatically, the possibility of errors is low, and exceeding of tolerance borders will be signalled immediately (Heeres and Vahl, 1997). In a liquid addition installation it is not common to dose and balance by hand; the installations are controlled automatically. It depends mainly on the accuracy of the installations if the right dosage is achieved within a range of tolerance.

Uniformity/homogeneity or distribution
The uniformity/homogeneity or distribution is usually evaluated by taking several samples from the bulk mixture and subsequently analysing the content of the targeted compound in each sample. The degree (or lack) of mixing is usually expressed as the variation or standard deviation of the measured values of key component content in the various samples, relative to the average content of the bulk mixture. This is often simplified to the coefficient of variation (Barendse, 1996; McCoy et al., 1994). Uniformity therefore can be measured by the coefficient of variation that is defined as:

$$CV = \frac{STD}{AVG} * 100 \qquad (2.1)$$

$$STD = \sqrt{\frac{n\sum x^2 - \left(\sum x\right)^2}{n^2}} \qquad (2.2)$$

where: CV   = coefficient of variation   [%]
          STD   = standard deviation   [-]
          AVG   = average or arithmetic mean   [-]
          n   = number of samples   [-]
          x   = value of one sample   [-]

Qualifying uniformity in terms of the coefficient of variation assumes a normal distribution. This is probably a very rough assumption, depending on the application. For example in spraying liquid additives on pellets a distribution as simplified by the thick line in figure 2.1 is very well possible. In any case for high variations of the average, a value of the additive level of $-10^{100}*AVG$ is not possible (less than 0), however, a value of $10^{100}*AVG$ is in theory possible.

At the moment, a definition of uniformity is missing in the GMP code. This definition is desirable in the future because a demand is made for uniformity of the number and size of the samples. The amount of the active component needs to have a coefficient of variation less than 5% for example. This value is partly dependent on the accuracy of the analysis. In many cases a coefficient of variation of 4% in the amount of active component, including analysis accuracy, is reachable (Heeres and Vahl, 1997). However, a coefficient of variation of 10% has become the accepted degree of variation separating uniform from non-uniform mixes (Beumer, 1991 and Wicker Poole, 1991).

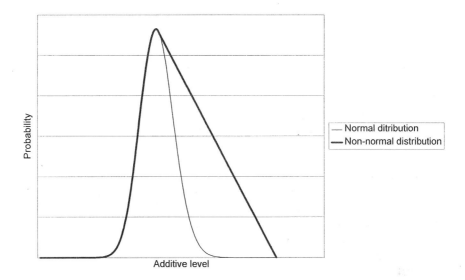

Figure 2.1 Normal distribution versus non-normal distribution.

Homogeneity and accuracy are strongly connected. They are both related to the right amount of additive being present in the feed. But where the accuracy of dosing is an indication of the average level of additive present, homogeneity is a measure of the variation around the average value. Additionally the scale at which the homogeneity is investigated is usually much smaller than that of the accuracy (Barendse, 1995). Another difference between the two is the fact that accuracy of dosing is usually concerned with keeping the amount of additive dosed in accordance with the volume of feed over distinct time intervals, for example batch runs, while homogeneity is a measure of variations over time as well as of spatial distribution of the additive over the feed. If variations are observed over large time intervals, this will influence both accuracy and homogeneity. Variations on a much smaller scale will only be visible in the measured homogeneity (Barendse, 1995). The coefficient of variation is therefore also dependent on the sample size as will be discussed in section 5.1. A smaller sample size will normally result in a higher coefficient of variation.

Carry-over
In a production installation the mash and fines that stay behind in the equipment after unloading generate carry-over. At the surface of an installation a cake of mash is formed. The amount of feed that stays in a mixer is increased when adding liquids in the mixer (Heeres and Vahl, 1997), see figure 2.2. The cake often exists of two layers: a relatively thick, caked layer, that stays for a longer time, and a relatively thin layer of light mash particles, that is replaced for every batch. The release of the thick cake gives an incidental carry-over. The thin layer of mash-particles gives a definite carry-over from every charge to the next charge. The area of the bunkers, transport and processing apparatus determine the amount of carry-over. Carry-over can be separated into carry-in and carry-out (Heeres and Vahl, 1997):

- Carry-out: the phenomenon that a part of the batch stays behind in the installation.
- Carry-in: the phenomenon that a part of the previous batch becomes part of the next batch.

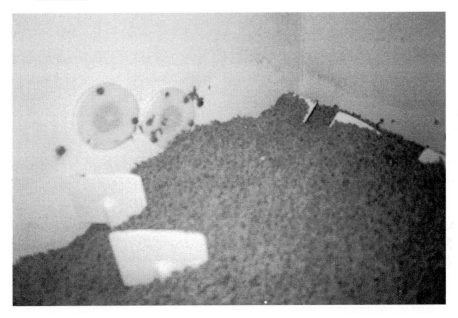

Figure 2.2 Sticking feed particles and dust with liquid to the sidewalls in a paddle mixer generating carry-over while adding 3 volume% liquid to piglet feed.

Reference: Engelen, 1998; unpublished

Contamination

Contamination is a form of carry-over, where active additives are carried over from previous batches to others. A part of the additives of a batch will run out with the next batch of feed and cause an undesirable component, which causes a different dosage or a 'pollution'. Contamination or 'pollution' of a feed can occur with (Heeres and Vahl, 1997; Schneider, 1998):

- Carry-in;
- Incidental loosening of the cake at the surface of the installation;
- Product derived from filters;
- Product derived from corners and gaps in the installation;
- Addition of for example returning feed.

The contamination of a single batch in a clean mixer can be measured by the recovery of an additive. This is the mean percentage of the total added additive that is found in the feed after analysing separate samples. The recovery can therefore be formulated according to equation 2.3:

$$RCV = \frac{AVG}{Dose\ level} *100 \qquad (2.3)$$

where: RCV   = recovery   [%]
        AVG   = average or arithmetic mean   [-]
        Dose level = dose level in same unit as average   [-]

2.2 QUALITY OF ANIMAL PRODUCTS

Certain feed additives contribute to improved quality of animal products, and their consumption has a direct effect on human health (Peisker, 1998). Examples of these are vitamin E, carotenoids and Ω-3 fatty acids. Hens' eggs for instance are ideal for enriching with vitamin E. If laying hen feed is enriched with vitamin E even at a level below 1000 IU per kg of feed (Table 2.1) one egg will contain enough of the vitamin to provide the recommended daily intake (12-15 mg) for an adult. Vitamin E also plays a special role in meat quality. Its property as an antioxidant means that it helps preserve the integrity of animal cells and prevents losses of cellular fluid (Peisker, 1998). The transfer rate in Table 2.1 is the percentage of available Vitamin E that is transferred from the feed into the egg.

Table 2.1 Transfer of vitamin E into the hens' eggs for different supplies of vitamin E.

Vitamin E addition [IU/kg feed]	Vitamin-E content [mg/egg]	Transfer rate [%]
0	1.1	37
100	3.7	23
1000	19.8	16
10000	35.3	3
20000	42.5	2

Reference: Peisker, 1998.

Carotenoids are used for the pigmentation of egg yolks and various types of seafood (e.g. salmon, trout, shrimps). They greatly increase the acceptance of these foods among consumers (Peisker, 1998).

Ω-3 fatty acids, known for their positive effect in preventing cardio-vascular disorders, are currently added to animal feed in the form of fish oils. Hens' eggs play a decisive role as accumulators of this substance. A certain proportion of these fatty acids must also be added to fish feed (Peisker, 1998).

3 LIQUID ADDITIVES

To produce feed of the lowest possible cost, the use of feed additives gives a useful contribution. In animal feeds, more and more additives are used (Harmanny according to Van Vliet, 1998). In order to get a better understanding of what is meant by an additive in this booklet, additives are defined as:

'materials that, when they are added in small amounts to the animal feed, can influence the production of the animals or the properties of the animal feed.'

However, animal feed additives have to meet with more demands. In relation to the health of the consumer, no harmful residues may be present in the animal products and the use may not lead to environmental pollution.

Additives are susceptible to degradation by environmental factors like extremes of pH, temperature, excessive friction and microbial growth. As an alternative to avoid micro-components undergoing the heat treatment, consideration should be given to adding the additives afterwards. It is then important to fix the additives to the pellet to prevent segregation in outloading, transport and storage and to prevent selection of different feed particles by the animal. The easiest way to fix the additive to the ready pellets or granules is by spraying liquid additives on the feed, where they are absorbed by the dry feed. Another possibility is sticking powder formulated additives on the granulates using a sticky liquid. This last technique, though not very easily applicable, gives the disadvantage that during attrition the additives will be separated from the pellets or granulates with the same consequences as not fixing the additives to the pellets, but only mixing them.

Some disadvantages of micro-components in powder form (Lucht, 1997) are:
- In the current technology micro-ingredients in powder form can only be added to mash formed mixtures, this means before the heat treatment or pelleting.
- With this mixing, segregation, forming of dust and contamination dangers are created. The dust formed from the micro-ingredients, forms a potential threat to the operation workers. The possible allergenic potential of some of the ingredients used, on the operating personnel, is considered to be especially disadvantageous with the common mixing and admixing processes, as these active ingredients may enter the breathing air and the skin in the form of dust (Abele, 1996).
- Micro-components that are added prior to a heat treatment need to be heat stable. This can be achieved for example by means of a coating. Normally a heat treatment causes considerable activity losses, which have to be compensated by an overdose, and increases feed costs.
- Micro-components in powder form often need to be mixed with a support material (carrier) in order to reach an amount that can be dosed.
- Micro-ingredients in powder form can be light flammable or explosive. In particular, the particle size and the humidity of a cloud of dust play an important role in this event. Fires and explosions are not exceptional in the compound industry (Harmanny according to Van Vliet, 1998).

In figure 3.1, some headlines are given for the use of powder or liquid based additive formulations. When using liquid based additive formulations this can be done in a post-pelleting application.

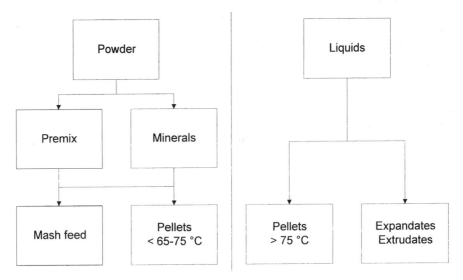

Figure 3.1 Headlines in the use of powder based or liquid based additive formulations, dependant on the process conditions.

Reference: Günther and Beudeker, 1997.

For an application with liquid additives the additive may need to be placed on a liquid carrier or to be mixed, to ensure the ability to spray. All mixtures need to be produced immediately prior to spraying, without significant storage of the liquid-mixture, to increase stability and therefore activity (Van der Poel, 1996).

Currently, wide ranges of dry micro-ingredients and premixes have liquid versions or analogues. These include amino acids, minerals, vitamins, enzymes, microbial products, flavours, organic acids and premixes. In the near future, certain antibiotics and growth promoters are likely to be available in liquid form (Gill, 1994). Vitamins, like many other micro-components, are usually produced in liquid form during chemical synthesis or fermentation and afterwards dried and put on a carrier (Schwarz, 1998a). If the additive is used in a liquid form these last two steps can be omitted and there is no need to ensure for stability against heat (Van der Poel, 1996; Schwarz, 1998a). The production of feed additives in the dry form can be a significant cost for products initially in liquid form and then dried or spray-dried on a carrier (Blair, 1996).

Converting additives to a powder product is currently done to make them easier to handle, to standardise the active substance content and to stabilise them against oxygen, moisture, pressure and trace elements with a pro-oxidative effect. Additionally, special processing stages during the formulation of some vitamins and carotenoids, such as micronisation to alter the primary particle size of the active substance, are intended to increase the bio-availability of the active substance (Schwarz, 1998a). Some advantages developing the dry form of additives will be lost if liquid formulation is desired for liquid addition.

Not all the additives are yet available in a fluid form, even enzymes. In particular, some highly functioning and widely used carbohydrases have, up to date been unavailable in a fluid form. According to one of the producers there is intensive research being carried out to get fluid formulations, but this needs time and will not be ready in the short run (Wagner, 1998).

Table 3.1 Micro-components that can be added in a liquid form.

Ingredient	Dose [g/tonne feed]
Enzymes (Single or mixes)	50-500
Amylases	
NSP enzymes	
Protease	
Phytases	50-100
Digestive enhancers	
Antibiotics	
Probiotics	500-5000
Prebiotics	
Vitamins	100-1000
Water soluble	
Fat soluble	
Medical basis	
Other additives	
Aromates	50-100
Colouring agents	
Antioxidants	50-500
Plant extracts	100-500
Amino acids	100-2000
Organic acids	3000-10000
Fat and Oil	

Reference: Lucht, 1997; Schwarz, 1998a.

Due to the often unpleasant taste of many active substances, the liquid formulation has to offer a high palatability (Van der Poel and Engelen, 1998). Besides that, problems in liquid additives can occur due to (Heidenreich, 1995):

- Difficulties in keeping the additives in solution (e.g. crystallisation);
- Liquid formulated additives do not have protection;
- Behaviour of suspensions of additives;
- Chemical compatibility of different additives and carrier liquids in comparison to stability in the contact time. This has to be examined separately in each case (Schwarz, 1998b).

3.1 NUTRITIVE ADDITIVES

Spraying of liquid additives also gives the possibility of adding vitamins and amino acids just before the transport of compound feed to the farmer (Van der Poel, 1996).

3.1.1 AMINO ACIDS

About 20 different amino acids are involved in building up body protein. The animal is unable to form some of these amino acids itself (essential amino acids). Consequently they have to be supplied in appropriate quantities via the feed (Limper, 1998). Knowledge of the quantitative amino-acid composition of raw materials is a main condition for the recipe of balanced compound feeds (except ruminants). A diet is optimal for protein when:

- The need of amino-acids of an animal specie (under given circumstances) is definitely covered;
- No amino-acids are available in abundance;
- It is the cheapest solution.

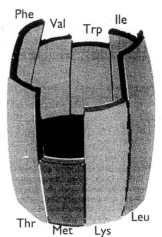

During protein synthesis, essential and non-essential amino acids are combined according to a pre-determined genetic code. To ensure that this process takes place continuously, all amino acids must be available in the body's amino acid pool. A shortage of non-essential amino acids can be compensated by transamination (transfer of nitrogen compounds), but if any one of the essential amino acids is missing, protein synthesis stops. The first amino acid (for poultry methionine, for pigs lysine) which interrupts protein synthesis in this way is called the first limiting amino acid in animal nutrition circles (Limper, 1998).

The model known as the 'Liebig barrel' demonstrates this concept (figure 3.2). Each stave of the barrel stands for one essential amino acid. The shortest stave determines the capacity of the barrel. If the shortest stave is lengthened (i.e. limiting amino acids are deliberately supplemented), the capacity of the protein synthesis can be raised to the level of the second

Figure 3.2 The Liebig barrel, each barrel stave represents one of the essential amino acids.

Reference: Limper, 1998.

limiting amino acid, and so on. The absolute limit of the protein forming capacity is genetically fixed. This explains why amino acids added above this boundary do not result in any further protein gain and have to be expelled again in the form of urea. It follows from the above that even adding small quantities of a limiting amino acid quite substantially increases the nutritive value of the feed (Limper, 1998). Normally amino acids are in a solid form, excluding lysine and methionine, which are often used in a liquid form.

3.1.2 *VITAMINS*

Most vitamins are used as an additive in small doses. Vitamins can also have a growth enhancing function (Rensink, 1998 and Whitehead, 1993). The most widely used and known vitamins for this purpose are vitamins A, B, C, D and E. In doses above the recommended dose, these all have a positive effect on the health if the circumstances are sub-optimal (Rensink, 1998).

Table 3.2 Impact of vitamins on the immune system.

Vitamin	Shortage	Supplementation
A	Reduced lymphocyte proliferation	Surplus toxic infections by enhancement of the intestine tissues and glands function.
β-Carotin	Increased risk of tumours	Stim. of T-lymphocytes, natural killer cells
B	Reduced lymphocyte proliferation and antibody production infections	Vitamin B_2, B_6, B_{12} and folic acid stimulate the immune function
C	Reduced phagocytosis	Positive influence on stress for humans, also for farm animals, that are constantly in a state of stress, further research could be useful; Improved immune function.
D		Promotes the function of the liver as a waste disposal and immunity builder.
E	Malfunction of T- and B-lymphocytes, natural killer cells and phagocytes	Antioxidant influences the protection in the cell membranes on unsaturated fats; Stim. cell division, positive effect on the reproduction organs; Stim. of T-lymphocytes, natural killer cells; Higher antibody titre.

Reference: Peisker, 1998; Rensink, 1998.

Feed manufacturers have a role in avoiding vitamin losses. No matter how well the manufacturers protect the vitamin products, the need to preserve bioavailability remains. The preparation of a mixture of trace minerals and vitamins, and the subsequent feed compounding processes are very aggressive and inevitably lead to some loss of vitamins. Each vitamin is affected by different factors so it is impossible to create a set of circumstances in feed compounding which is acceptable to all products (Putnam and Taylor, 1997).

Chapter 3

Factors that can affect the stability of vitamins are (Putnam and Taylor, 1997):

- Temperature: Increased temperatures affect many vitamins. Most vitamins are at their most stable between 5 and 10°C.
- Water/humidity: frequently accelerates oxidation. In some cases water vapour is more aggressive, in others water droplets can be destructive. These features can be accelerated by increased temperature.
- Acidity/alkalinity: The pH of a mixture can have a marked effect on vitamin stability. Most are affected by extremes of pH (<3 or >11), many are unstable at pH 3-5 and one or two between pH 5-8. This leaves the most stable range at pH 5-8.
- Oxygen: most vitamins are destroyed by oxidation, they can be affected by oxygen in the air and by oxidising agents.
- Light: UV light and other forms of radiation (e.g. gamma irradiation for sterilisation) can destroy many vitamins.
- Trace minerals: Many trace mineral ions catalyse the various processes which can destroy vitamins. For example, copper and iron ions act as catalysts in oxidation, while oxides and hydroxides of metals produce an alkaline pH.
- Physical effects: Physical action of hammers in a mill can pulverise protected beadlets exposing the vitamin. During extrusion, the pressure used to push the feed through the extruder generates a very high friction temperature, which can destroy heat-sensitive vitamins.
- Storage time: most of the destructive effects are time related: the longer the premix or feed is stored, the greater the loss of vitamin activity.

Table 3.3 Factors influencing the stability of pure vitamins.

Vitamin	Tempera-ture	Oxygen	Water	Light	Acid	Alkali	Retention [%][a]
A	**	**	*	**	*	0	80
D$_3$	*	**	*	*	*	0	75
E	0	0	*	*	0	**	80
K$_3$	*	*	**	0	**	0	20
B$_1$	*	*	**	0	0	**	90
B$_2$	0	0	*	**	0	0	95
B$_6$	**	0	*	*	*	0	95
B$_{12}$	**	*	*	*	0	0	95
Calcium pantothenate (B$_3$)	*	0	*	0	*	0	95
Niacin	0	0	0	0	0	0	95
Folic acid	**	0	**	**	**	0	95
Biotin	*	0	0	0	0	0	95
C	0	**	**	0	0	*	25

0 = stable, * = sensitive, ** = very sensitive.
[a]   Stability of vitamins after expanding and a storage time of two months
Reference: Putnam and Taylor, 1997; Albers, 1996.

Table 3.3 shows how the individual vitamins are affected by the major destructive factors. The most stable is Niacin (Nicotinic acid or Nicotinamide), which is hardly affected by any of these influences. At the other end of the spectrum, folic acid, vitamin K (as K3 analogues) and vitamin C (as crystalline ascorbic acid) are seriously affected by several factors which can combine with time to destroy a large proportion of these present in a feed or premix. Schwarz (1998) found similar results compared to Albers (1996) with fish-feed and extrusion. The destructive effects of the various factors listed relate to the pure vitamin material before it is given any form of protective coating. Coatings and other forms of protection reduce but cannot entirely prevent losses of activity because of the need to preserve bioavailability (Putnam and Taylor, 1997). Rather than formulating a premix by determining an appropriate amount of each vitamin from tables of allowances, it may be better to work out how much should be in the feed when it is eaten by the animal, and working backwards taking the losses at each stage of the process into account, so an overdose will be necessary (Putnam and Taylor, 1997).

3.2   NON NUTRITIVE ADDITIVES OR GUT FLORA STABILISERS

3.2.1   ENZYMES

The predominant ingredients in animal feed formulations are of plant origin. Plant material is known to contain many compounds, which are inefficiently utilised by economically important monogastric animals such as pigs and poultry (Van Dijck and Geerse, 1993). Addition of enzymes to diets for monogastric animals is now an established practice, particularly in young animals, growing poultry and to a lesser extent growing and fattening pigs (Perry, 1997). Enzymes are of essential importance in the pre-digestion of an animal. Classified in large categories we distinguish proteases, lipases and carbohydrate cleaving enzymes, like amylases, which as bio-catalysts have the task of degrading feed components to a form that is readily absorbed by the animal. The main compounds hampering optimal feed utilisation in this respect are dietary fibre, also termed non-starch polysaccharides (NSP), and antinutritional factors (ANF) comprising a variety of structurally different components, such as trypsin inhibitors, phytate and tannins or other polyphenolic structures. The effects of the presence of these compounds in feed ingredients can be minimised by either technological processing, for example toasting or extrusion, or by supplementation with microbial enzymes (Van Dijck and Geerse, 1993). The potential of enzymes (Table 3.4) is determined by the improvement or increase of the ME (Metabolisable energy) of raw materials (Van der Ploeg, 1989).

Table 3.4 Currently available thermo-stable enzymes and their applications.

Enzyme	Process Temperature	Application
Carbohydrases		
α-Amylase (bacterial)	9-110	Starch hydrolysis, brewing, baking, textiles
α-Amylase (fungal)	50-60	Maltose
β-Glucanase		Barley containing feeds
Xylanase		Wheat containing feeds
Pentosanase		Rye containing feeds
Oligosaccharidases		Short chain carbohydrates
Phytase		Breakdown of plant phytate, a major form of plant phosphorous
Glucoamylase	50-60	Maltodextrin hydrolysis
Pullanase	5-60	High glucose syrups
Xylose isomerase	50-60	High fructose syrups
β-Galactosidase	30-50	Lactose hydrolysis
Cellulase	45-60	Cellulose hydrolysis
Pectinase	30-50	Clarification of fruit juices
Proteases		
Acid proteases	30-50	Food processing
Neutral proteases (fungal)	40-60	Baking, brewing
Alkaline proteases	40-60	Detergents
Lipases	30-70	Detergents, food processing

Reference: Perry, 1997; Campbell and Bedford, 1992.

For more details in the principles and working mechanisms of the various enzymes, the reader is referred to the papers of Campbell and Bedford (1992) and Van Dijck and Geerse (1993).

The effect of the use of enzymes in compound feeds can be seen from practical experiments (e.g. Van der Ploeg, 1989: Table 3.5). In this booklet the results of one of the trials will be shown to overview the effect of the enzyme product Porzyme SP® in a normal weaned pig feed with an EW=1.10 and an available lysine content of 1.08%. The experimental feed only differed in the addition of 0.1% Porzyme-SP®, see Table 3.5. The weaning age was 3 weeks and the experiment lasted 7 weeks.

Table 3.5 Two practical trials in Belgium with Porzyme-SP®.

	Control	Control + enzyme
Farm 1 (Belgium landrace)		
Number of pigs	27	27
Repeats	3	3
Start weight [kg] [%]	5.6 [100]	5.7 [100]
End weight [kg]	17.8	19.6
Weight gain [g/day] [%]	238 [100]	273 [115]
Feed intake [g/day] [%]	464 [100]	510 [110]
Feed gain [-] [%]	1.95 [100]	1.87 [96]
Farm 2 (Belgium landrace * Pietrain)		
Number of pigs	26	27
Repeats	3	3
Start weight [kg] [%]	6.3 [100]	6.2 [98]
End weight [kg]	20.5	20.6
Weight gain [g/day] [%]	254 [100]	257 [101]
Feed intake [g/day] [%]	472 [100]	445 [94]
Feed gain [-] [%]	1.86 [100]	1.73 [94]

Reference: Van der Ploeg, 1989.

Due to their high efficiency the addition of enzymes is often in only small amounts. For example the liquid phytase form (Natuphos® 5000 L) requires doses of 60-120 g/tonne, liquid forms of NSP-splicing enzymes (Natugrain® 33% L) require 225-300 g/tonne. This is respectively 50-100 ml phytase and 195-260 ml NSP-splicing enzyme (Günther and Beudeker, 1997).

Enzymes, like all other proteins, are susceptible to degradation by environmental factors like extremes of pH, temperature, excessive friction, microbial growth and a range of others. As a general rule it can be stated that all these processes proceed faster at elevated temperatures as well as with high(er) water activities (Van Dijck and Geerse, 1993). Although stability enhancements can and have been made by means of protein engineering and formulation measures, basically nature defines the possibilities (Barendse, 1995). The compound industry is involved with high temperature processes and the application of enzymes. Important factors in these are the height of the temperature, the duration of the process and the humidity content of the feed. In an extended process line, higher temperature and humidity content of the feed cause higher enzyme destruction (Günther and Beudeker, 1997) by denaturation and the enzymes will be inactivated (Barendse and Van Doessum, 1993).

Activity losses of stabilised additives during thermal processing cannot be avoided but must be minimised by the control of process conditions (and its variation) during routine feed manufacturing (Van der Poel and Engelen, 1998). Studies with a wide range of fungal enzymes revealed that without protection, in feed, activity was rapidly lost at conditioning feed temperatures of 60 °C. Granular enzymes where substrate stabilisation occurred, could be used up to 75 °C and coating of the granules allowed conditioning temperatures of the feed up to 80 °C to be applied. Bacterial enzymes, for example, were more heat stable than those from fungi and some could tolerate 85 to 90 °C for short periods (Cowan, 1993).

Enzyme stability during feed processing is difficult to establish in the laboratory. Firstly the levels of enzyme activities in feeds are very low and secondly, quantitative analysis is often problematic due to strong binding of the enzymes to feed, which prevents complete enzyme extraction prior to assay. However, it has been established that measuring gut viscosity of broilers can be used to estimate enzyme activity in the intestinal tract (Bedford et al., 1992).

A trial was conducted with an enzyme product stabilised onto a cereal substrate carrier to test the effect of preconditioning and pelleting temperature on stability of the product. The barley based (602 g/kg) feed together with the dry enzyme product was preconditioned for 30 seconds at 75, 85 and 95 °C followed by pelleting and fed to chicks from 1 to 19 days of age with six replicates per diet. Results from the trial are summarised in Table 3.6.

Table 3.6 Effect of enzyme addition on digesta viscosity and performance in chicks fed from 1 – 19 days of age pelleted diets conditioned at 75, 85 or 95 °C.

Conditioning temperature [°C]	Diet	Digesta viscosity [cPs]	Weight gain [g]	Feed gain
75	Control	26.8[a]	544[ab]	1.64[ab]
75	+ Enzyme	4.6[b]	562[ab]	1.52[b]
85	Control	20.7[b]	556[ab]	1.60[ab]
85	+ Enzyme	6.1[b]	561[b]	1.50[b]
95	Control	30.6[a]	482[ab]	1.75[ab]
95	+ Enzyme	8.7[b]	510[ab]	1.68[ab]

Avizyme SX®, FFI, UK
[ab] Means not sharing a common superscript differ significantly (p<0.05)
Reference: Peisker, 1993.

Effects and interaction of expander processing and enzymes were studied in a trial. Broiler diets containing 603 g/kg wheat and 200 g/kg soyabean-meal were either pelleted or expanded and pelleted, and supplemented with dry or liquid enzymes. The diets were produced at the pilot plant of Amandus Kahl Nachf., Reinbek, Germany with the following processing conditions:

- Pelleted feeds (mash preconditioning at 60 °C and 15% moisture for 30 seconds, expander by-passed, pellet temperature at press outlet 75 °C);
- Expanded feeds (mash preconditioning at 60 °C and 15% moisture for 30 seconds, expanding at 17% moisture and temperature 105 °C prior to outlet, expander temperature at the outlet 95 °C, pellet temperature at press outlet 75 °C).

After pelleting the three millimetre pellets were cooled in a horizontal cooler to 25 °C. Liquid enzyme was sprayed homogeneously onto the pellets after cooling in a special batch mixer. The experimental diets were fed to six groups of 24 chicks per group from seven to 28 days of age. Results from gut viscosity, feed intake and live weight gain measurements are presented in Table 3.7.

Table 3.7 Effect of enzyme addition in dry (mixed pre-pelleting) or liquid (sprayed pelleting) from pre or post-pelleting on performance (7-28 days) and gut digesta viscosity in broilers at 21 days.

Diet 7-28 days [g]	Digesta viscosity [cPs]	Weight gain 21 d [g]	Feed gain
Pelleted control	6.9[a]	1155[ab]	1.50[a]
Pelleted + dry enzyme	4.3[b]	1173[a]	1.47[ab]
Pelleted + liquid enzyme	4.0[b]	1158[ab]	1.47[ab]
Expanded/pelleted control	20.0[c]	1124[b]	1.53[a]
Exp./pell. + liquid enzyme	3.8[b]	1177[a]	1.39[b]

Avizyme TX®, FFI, UK
[a-c]   Means not sharing a common superscript differ significantly (p<0.05)
Reference: Liebert et al., 1993.

The effectiveness of, for example, carbohydrases included in high-temperature pellets is also reflected in broiler studies on small-scale and production level by Gadient et al. (1994). When carbohydrase was added in the dry form to mash feed, a close relationship was found in the pellets between enzyme level (xylanase) and pelleting temperature, see figure 3.3. The same pattern can be seen in animal performance (Gadient et al., 1994). Obviously, the critical temperature for this particular enzyme stability is around 75-80 °C. The use of the liquid form of this enzyme reflected that animal performance was up to the level of the feed pelleted below the critical temperature.

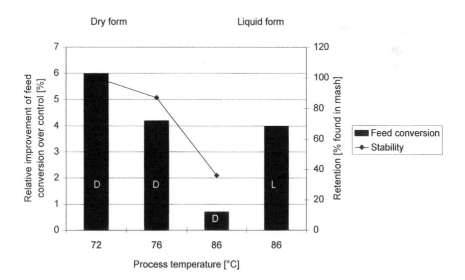

Figure 3.3 Enzyme stability and broiler performance, depending on pelleting temperature of feed and the form of carbohydrase-enzyme.

Reference: Gadient et al., 1994.

Enzymes are biological catalysts, which are temperature sensitive like all other proteins. Even when data during conditioning or pelleting, expansion or extrusion are known it is still hard to predict the stability of enzymes during compound production. The determination of the stability of enzymes can only take place on the spot (Günther and Beudeker, 1997). In liquid form enzyme stability can be improved by addition of, for example, salts and sugars to lower the water activity of the liquid. Another way of stabilising enzymes is to remove most of the water by drying to produce dry enzyme concentrates. Dry enzymes have superior storage stability over their liquid counterparts. Dry products are often easier to mix homogeneously into feeds than liquids (Nissinen, 1994; Günther and Beudeker, 1997).

Mixes of liquid phytase with water (1:10) are sufficiently stable in a 24-hour storage. In practice it is, however, recommended to use diluted phytase without intermediate storage to prevent microbial contamination (Günther and Beudeker, 1997). After spraying of the liquid enzymes on the feed pellets, the enzymes are relatively stable during storage. This is caused by the lower water activity in the feed. After storage of the feed for three months at 20 and 30 °C, a phytase activity of ± 85% is found. Coating of the feed pellets with fat or oil does not increase the stability (Günther and Beudeker, 1997).

In a trial to mix some competing products with a mixture of phytase from Natuphos liquid® the results in figure 3.4 were found. Whereas, in another trial a mixture of Natuphos liquid® and an NSP enzyme preparation gave no negative effect on the enzyme activity within eight days (Schwarz, 1998b).

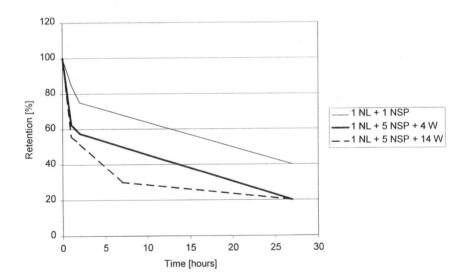

Figure 3.4 Stability of Natuphos liquid® (NL) in mixtures with a NSP-degrading enzyme (NSP) and water (W).

Reference: Schwarz, 1998b.

In mixtures with choline chloride and glycerine, at least 95% of the added phytase activity was found even 24 hours after the mixture was made. In contrast, dramatic losses of enzymes are observed right form the beginning when propionic acid and propylene glycol are used. Even where ammonia propionate with a comparatively moderate pH value of about 6 was used, roughly one third of the activity was lost within a short time. Here too, no residual activity is found after 24 hours of storage at room temperature, see Table 3.8 (Schwarz, 1998b)

Table 3.8 Compatibility of phytase (from Natuphos liquid®) with various liquid feedstuffs/feed additives.

Feedstuff/Feed additive	Mixing ratio	Appearance	Retention after hours [% of analysed content]		
			0	2.5	24
Choline chloride 75	1+5	Transparent	99	97	97
Propionic acid	1+9	Precipitation/phase separation	23	22	0
Ammonium propianate	1+9	Transparent	66	69	0
Propandiol	1+9	Transparent, after approximately 24 h. cloudy	41	40	0
Soybean oil	1+9	Emulsion, immediate phase separation	-	-	-
Glycerol	1+9	transparent	88	94	95

Reference: Schwarz, 1998b.

3.2.2 ANTIBIOTICS

Feeds containing pharmacologically active substances are used for the purposes of therapy. The process for the production of feed also includes feed containing pharmacologically active feed additives, in particular, antibiotic and non-antibiotic performance enhancing products (feed saving), as well as additives for the prevention of diseases (Abele, 1996). Feed additives with pharmacological action are mixed into the feed in accordance with their application as prescribed by regulation.

For experts there is no question that the development towards more concentrated and intensive animal production necessarily provokes more stress and diseases. For that reason, on the one hand, there is no doubt of an increasing need for medicated feed for the purpose of therapy as well as for additives for the prevention of diseases (Abele, 1996). On the other hand though, consumer and politicians do not think that antibiotics have a (standard) place in animal feeds, especially for resistance of phatogens for antibiotics in humans as well as animals (Rensink, 1998; Van den Boogaard, 1998; Nijland, 1998). The compound feed industry is already developing and thinking of ways to get round a possible ban of antibiotic-like digestive enhancers mainly in the areas of alternatives such as probiotics and prebiotics. In Denmark, the use of antimicrobial and chemotherapeutic growth promoters is prohibited not by law but more or less by society since March 1998 in feeds for pigs up 35 kilograms (Makkink, 1998; Anonymous, 1998b). In Sweden, the use of antibiotics as a growth promoter has been prohibited since 1986

(Van den Boogaard, 1998), however they may have to allow antibiotics again due to European Union politics, if the EU does not prohibit antibiotics in feeds itself (Anonymous, 1998b).

Cross-contamination and residues

The whole process of mixing, conveying, pelleting, lifting, cooling and storing facilities carries over considerable amounts of pharmacologically active substances into subsequent batches of feed. These carried-over drugs and feed additives contaminate subsequent batches and may result in undesirable interaction between the different pharmacological components of the batches involved. Feeding these contaminated feeds conceals the danger of considerable residue problems in the production of animal feeds (Abele, 1996). To avoid these problems at least two cleaning batches should be conveyed through the feed production facilities. This procedure however is not very economical nor does it solve the actual problem, as it immediately raises the question of what to do with the cleaning batches.

Applying pharmacologically active substances downstream from pelleting in a PPA application consists in applying certain antibiotics, anthelmintics, coccidiostatics and growth promoters in liquid form using a spraying system can avoid these problems. Liquid forms of medicated premixes for calves, cows, beef cattle, pigs, piglets and fish are available (Abele, 1996).

Requirements for a medicated premix in liquid form (Abele, 1996):
1. It must conform to licensing requirements, and is subject to the regulations as prescribed by the licensing authorities.
2. The pharmacologically active substances in liquid form must be stable under the following conditions:
   a) The substances as such must be stable in the liquid for at least one year and after spray-application on the feed for not less than two months.
   b) As the majority of those substances cannot be dissolved in the liquid carrier in the desired concentrations, it is necessary to formulate homogeneous and stable suspensions.
   c) Formulations also have to be stable with regard to microbiology.
3. Formulations should have the ability to adhere to the feed pellets.
4. Due to the bitter and unpleasant taste of many active substances, the liquid formulation has to offer a high palatability.

Generally these formulations are non-aqueous thixotrophic gels containing active substances at levels of 10 to 30%. The thixotrophic character prevents sedimentation of the mostly non-dissolved ingredients and assures a homogeneous suspension. These gels can be pumped on to the spraying equipment (Abele, 1996; Peisker, 1995).

3.2.3 PROBIOTICS

Probiotics are often seen as an alternative for antibiotics as performance enhancers. Therefore the market for probiotics is expected to increase in the near future (Wagner, 1998). It can be ascertained that probiotics will lead to clear securing of higher performance, according to various trials, for example those published by Kühn (1998). Probiotics can be separated into lactic acid producing bacteria, Bacillus spores and yeasts (Rensink, 1998; Kühn, 1998). Probiotics as a group of live micro-organisms go through the same exposure as for example pathogenic micro-organisms in hydrothermal processes and lose their activity (Peisker, 1995). In some cases only temperatures of 65 °C can be tolerated. Sometimes, in an encapsulated form, temperatures from 85 to 90 °C are possible. For heat treatment in this encapsulated form this means globally: 'pelleting is possible, expanding and extruding is not possible' (Wagner, 1998).

Lactic acid producing bacteria
Naturally lactic acid producing bacteria are present in the intestine flora in great numbers. An addition of extra strong, more productive groups can reduce the number of other bacteria by a decreasing pH and an occupation of the intestine surface (competitive exclusion). Lactic acid producing bacteria can also prevent the affixation of other germs to the intestinal surface by the secretion of defined fluids (Rensink, 1998).

Bacillus spores
Different species are used in animal feeds. Bacillus spores form enzymes in the intestine that have a negative effect on the bacteria growth in the intestine (Kühn, 1998). Also an immunising effect is ascribed to these Bacillus spores (Rensink, 1998).

Yeasts
Yeasts are used in monogastric as well as in ruminant feeds. In ruminants, the positive effect is based on stabilising the pH in the rumen, which reduces the possibilities of an acidose. The microbial transformation of the nutrients therefore is more efficient and the performance enhanced. For monogastric animals, the yeasts may cause a reduction in the number of coli-species. On the one hand yeasts have the capability of binding the coli-species and their metabolism products (enterotoxines), and on the other hand they prevent the affixation of the coli-species to the intestinal surface. Moreover, yeasts produce substances that promote the metabolism of their host (Rensink, 1998).

Induced by their specific working mechanisms probiotics will have to be supplied to the animal on a daily basis in constant quantities (Rensink, 1998). Most probiotics can nowadays be formulated as a liquid. Therefore a special gel is used; this overcomes separation during transport and storage. The gels are not harmful for the animal and can technologically be seen as a fluid (Peisker, 1995). The physical properties of these gels are significantly different from water solutions and can be characterised with the definition (thixotrop). That means that the flow characteristics change with an increasing loss of shear (Peisker, 1995).

Not all probiotics are presently available in a fluid form as a suspension or an emulsion. There is still little information available regarding the compliance with other additives (Wagner, 1998).

3.2.4 PREBIOTICS

Prebiotics are substances that work as food for the micro-organisms in the alimentary tract. Prebiotics are not intended to be metabolised by the host. Selective distribution gives the possibility to adjust the composition of the micro flora. For example NDOs (Non-digestible oligosacchharides) have a purpose as feed for certain lactobacilli that push away harmful organisms. Mannanoligosaccharides (MOS) for example can bind coli-species and remove them from the host intestines (Rensink, 1998).

3.3 REQUIREMENTS FOR DIET COMPOSITION

To achieve a well-balanced feed, a number of important points regarding additives can be described:
1. Under or Overdose of additives;
2. Diluting of additives/water activity;
3. Adding and mixing of multiple additives;
4. Pellet size.

Under or Overdose of additives
The importance of the accuracy of dosing is clear: a too low overall addition level would decrease the effect of the additive and thereby damage the quality of the feed, too high a dosage level would be generally unacceptable from an economic point of view as the components under consideration are usually of a high value (Barendse, 1995). An overdose also leads in some situations to a reduced efficacy (Harker, 1995). An overdose can, for example, lead to digestion of the body's own tissues. The implications of inaccurate dosing are translated to the economic performance of broilers by Harker (1995). He found a clear dose-response relationship that existed between the enzyme dose and the broiler performance, see figure 3.5.

Harker (1995) found that a shortage as well as an overdose of enzyme has a negative effect on the feed cost response (FCR), this can also be showed in a theoretical effect where the relationship between the recovery, coefficient of variation and the dose rate is illustrated (figure 3.6) (Harker, 1995).

Figure 3.6 gives a statistical illustration of the effect of poor enzyme dosing accuracy on the distribution of enzyme between samples within a batch ('population') of feed. For the purpose of this illustration the target dose rate is assumed to be 0.5 kg/tonne feed. Dosing accuracy is measured in terms of mean recovery (RCV) and coefficient of variation (CV) of enzyme activity from samples within a batch of feed (Harker, 1995).

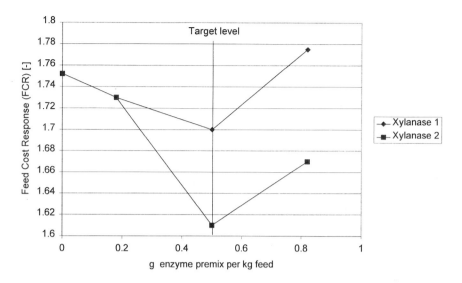

Figure 3.5 Dose response of broilers to 2 different xylanases from Tichoderma.
10 replicates of 7 broilers per diet, 0-21 days, 49% wheat, 15% triticale.

After: Harker, 1995.

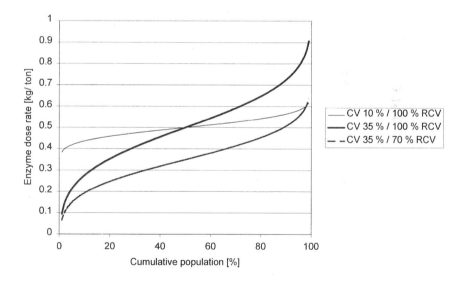

Figure 3.6 Theoretical effect of 3 different levels of dosing accuracy (expressed as
% coefficient of variation (CV) and % recovery in a normal distribution) on dose
rate (g/tonne of feed) assuming a target dose rate of 0.5 kg/tonne.

After: Harker, 1995.

The CV 35%/RCV 70% -line in figure 3.6 represents a low accuracy level in which 25% of the feed samples contain less than 0.3 kg/tonne i.e. < 60% of target enzyme activity. Reference to the dose response relationship described earlier (figure 3.5) indicates that 0.3 kg/tonne would have reduced feed cost response by at least 30-60% (0.02-0.08 points) in that study (Harker, 1995). CV 35%/RCV 100% also represents a poor level of dosing accuracy, in contrast CV 10%/RCV 100% represents a high degree of dosing accuracy with very few samples of feed receiving enzyme dose levels above or below the target, thereby ensuring a consistent and cost effective response to the enzyme (Harker, 1995). It is evident that the level of additive present in separate portions of the feed should always be sufficiently close to the target level to obtain the desired effect (Barendse, 1995). The experimental found-values of additives should not exceed 10% more or less than the desired value (Heidenreich, 1998).

In contrast to the above arguments a trade-off between accuracy and homogeneity might be economically interesting. When the volumes of feed being treated with PPA are comparatively low, the investment in a high-tech installation might not be feasible. A process yielding a product of relatively low homogeneity might be installed. Appropriate levels of the additive in a sufficient percentage of the samples can be achieved by raising the overall dosage of the additive. Of course this only applies to additives which can be overdosed without harmful effects to the target animals (Barendse, 1995; Barendse and Van Doesum, 1993). In figure 3.7, the influence of the homogeneity of an additive in a feed mix in order to guarantee the required dose in a daily ration of an animal is reflected (Barendse and Van Doesum, 1993).

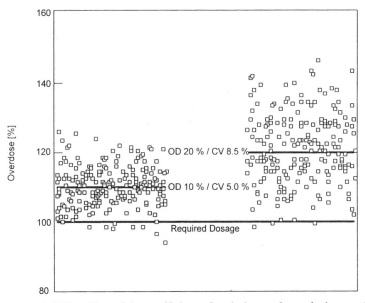

Figure 3.7 The effect of the coefficient of variation and overdosing on the achieve of the desired dosage in a daily ration of an animal.

OD = overdose, CV = coefficient of variation

After: Barendse and Van Doesum, 1993.

In figure 3.8, the possibility of a shortage of additive for the animal can be seen in the relationship of the coefficient of variation and the overdose. This figure shows that samples with a shortage of additive are inevitable. This applies for every component in a mixture (Barendse and Van Doesum, 1993). The graphs in figure 3.8 are simulated on the assumption that the measured content is normally distributed in the feed. Therefore it is clear that with an overdose of 0% there is a 50:50 chance of finding a shortage and at the same time a 50:50 chance of finding an overdose. It is also clear that if the coefficient of variation is 10%, the possibility of an animal getting, in the two following days, a ration with a shortage of 10% is then 3.6%. For the three following days this possibility will be less than 0.5%.

Comparing both the graphs of the model-study in figure 3.8 shows if a chance of 10% on a shortage of 15% is acceptable, so 90% of the measurements are greater than 85% of the desired value, this can be achieved with an overdose of 0% at a coefficient of variation of 10% or with an overdose of about 15% at a coefficient of variation of 20%.

Diluting of additives/water activity
The very low concentration that is required of liquid additives requires very precise equipment and controls. It then seems logical to dilute additives with water or oil, for example, and also to increase the number of droplets which will have a positive effect on the additive distribution (Van der Poel and Engelen, 1998).

The dilution, however, should be limited in view of negative effects on pellet quality (hardness and durability) and of microbial decay (Barendse, 1993). Diluting increases the water activity. It can thus be compulsory by law to make pre-mixes of fluids (dilutions) while minimal doses of feed additives can be prescribed (Günther and Beudeker, 1997). In practice diluting is used to increase the accuracy of the installation (Van Leeuwen, 1998; Günther and Beudeker, 1997).

The water activity (a_w) or equilibrium relative humidity is defined as the relative humidity generated at equilibrium by a product in a closed system at constant temperature (Sneider and Betz, 1991). This can be described in a formula as in equation 3.1.

$$a_w = \frac{p}{ps}$$
(3.1)

where: a_w = Water activity [-]
p = Water pressure above the surface of the sample material [-]
ps = Water pressure above the surface of pure water at the same temperature [-]

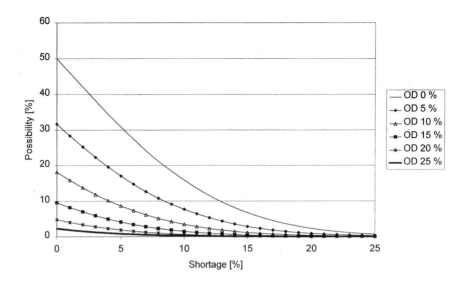

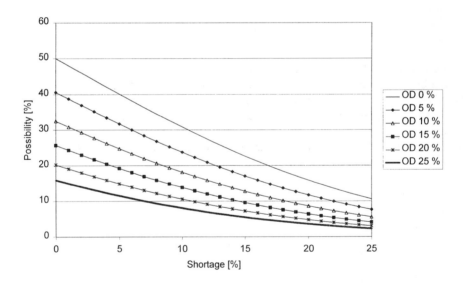

Figure 3.8 The effect of an overdose on the possibility to find one sample, the size of a daily ration, with less additive than desired with a coefficient of variation equalling 10% in the upper figure and equalling 20% in the lower figure.

OD = overdose

After: Barendse and Van Doesum, 1993.

Samples may retain water by chemical bonding, absorption by surface phenomena, capillary condensation and formation of a solution. Depending on the nature of the material and its water content, several of these factors may contribute to the equilibrium relative humidity. Strongly bound water is practically unavailable; the water activity is low. However, 'free' water will show high water activity. This free water is measured as a_w without definition of its origin and amount present (Sneider and Betz, 1991).

Because 'free' water is available for chemical reactions and biological processes, the water activity has gained significance in the food and feed industry for predicting microbial stability.

Table 3.9 Limits of growth in micro-organisms as a function of the water activity.

Water activity (a_w)	Microbiological type
0.91-0.95	Most bacteria
0.88	Yeast fungi
0.8	Most moulds
0.75	Halophilic bacteria
0.7	Osmophilic bacteria
0.65	Xerophilic moulds

Reference: Sneider and Betz, 1991.

As a rule of thumb, a limit value of $a_w = 0.65$ (25 °C) must not be exceeded in order to prevent microbial growth (Sneider and Betz, 1991). If the water activity limit is exceeded, the feeds must be protected by preservatives, for example propionic acid. However, even in cases where the a_w is below 0.65, it must be considered that during storage the water content can be locally higher, due to the influence of heat and moisture condensation in silos. The determination of water activity is a valuable tool in the prediction of microbial stability of feeds.

Adding and mixing of multiple additives
In principle it is possible to spray one or more fluids in a PPA-installation. In practice, to add multiple additives, a mixture is often made (Van Leeuwen, 1998). It is urgently recommended to dose liquid enzymes/additives alone. In single (non-mixed) form spraying, it is possible to spray the additive directly out of the original storage onto the feed. The danger of bacterial contamination with other additives and negative effects for the stability are then minimised (Günther and Beudeker, 1997). The enzymes are not compliant with acids, other liquid additives and carrier liquids (Heidenreich, 1995). If possible, contact with liquid fats and melasses should be prevented. All these contacts decrease the activity rapidly (Wagner, 1998). Also physical compatibility should be recognised in that two combined enzymes may result for example in foaming (Van der Poel and Engelen, 1998).

Chapter 3

Pellet size
Several mechanisms play a role where pellet size is concerned. An increase in pellet size means that there are fewer pellets in the same sample weight. Additionally, when the feed pellets are coarser, it will become more difficult to reach the optimal independent distribution of liquid over the feed. These mechanisms will reduce homogeneity when pellet size increases (Barendse, 1995). Due to the increased size it is thus easier to spray a larger fraction in a given volume of feed pellets during the PPA process and this in most cases will compensate for the previously mentioned effects. Since the coefficient of variation is more strongly dependent on fraction sprayed pellets than on sample size and variation due to distribution of the liquid over the sprayed feed will in most cases be only a minor contribution to the total variation, one would even expect that larger feed pellets would give a better homogeneity assuming use of the same equipment, identical sample sizes and virtually complete mixing (Barendse, 1995).

Other requirements
Since animals with small daily rations are usually fed smaller pellets, the PPA processing of these feeds require extra attention. The small daily rations and the possible reduction of hit fraction according to the above considerations make it harder to reach the desired levels of homogeneity (Barendse, 1995).

4 PPA-EQUIPMENT

In overviewing the dosing of contamination sensitive additives such as pharmacologically active products, enzymes and probiotics, there are particular advantages for the compound feed industry in using post-pelleting applications (Peisker, 1995):

- no extra product line for medical feed preparation;
- no cross-contamination;
- no problems with remaining feed in equipment;
- no 'wash' charges;
- no loss in active product;
- higher security for the labourers.

For the farmer it means the highest possible precision in therapy and probiotics and no danger of parts of previous batches in the normal feed (Peisker, 1995).

As mentioned before, it is not easy to add precise amounts of a liquid to a dry feed mixture. If the liquid is poured into the mixer, it often fails to disperse. If it is sprayed into the mixer, the spray nozzles may clog or the mixing tools become coated. If it is combined with other liquids in a liquid premix, it may interact and become unstable or degrade. If the liquid is sticky or electrostatic, dangerous residues may be deposited downstream throughout the production system. Moreover, simply measuring some liquids can be problematic as temperature may affect their density and hence the accuracy of flow-type metering devices (Gill, 1994). Additives can be sprayed as liquids on pellets and granulates in an undiluted formula in small amounts with the help of available equipment. It results in better quality to spray on an *equally sized* granulate as expandate or extrudate than on a pelleted feed with fines (Wagner, 1998)

While choosing an appropriate mixing system for liquid additives attention needs to be paid to the desired dosage accuracy, e.g. 0.002 to 1.0%, and the uniformity of the distribution of the additives in the feed (Barendse and Van Doesum, 1993). In principle there is a choice between an advanced system that guarantees a high accuracy and uniformity, and a cheaper, simpler system with a lack of accuracy and uniformity, that can be corrected by a higher additive dosage. This is a wide range to choose from, and the best system will be a compromise between these two extremes (Van der Poel, 1996). In the application of oliogels, the choice between pumps, tubes, and valves is more important than for water or oily fluids. These gels give the opportunity to create different pharmaceutically active products as well as performance enhancers as a fluid additive (Peisker, 1995).

Several suppliers have entered the market with post-processing liquid application equipment. Some, designed primarily for fat addition, have been adapted for micro liquids. Other systems have been designed for dedicated application of certain types of micro liquids, such as enzymes. However, a number of systems have demonstrated flexibility in the variety and amount of micro liquids they can apply (Gill, 1994).

Chapter 4

4.1 POSITIONING LIQUID ADDITION IN THE PRODUCTION LINE

When we look at the process in a compound factory schematically, then the raw materials are processed firstly in a mash compound feed. This mash-feed is either pelleted, extruded or expanded afterwards. Addition of liquids in the main mash mixer is not an option. The build-up of agglomerates and left-over feed on the surfaces in the form of crusts and burn will increase the carry-over and cross contamination, and cannot even be removed by a rinse charge (Heidenreich, 1998).

At the exit of the pellet press, extruder or expander, fat or oil is often added. This position is in one respect ideal for adding liquid additives because the pellets are still weak, porous and therefore have a high absorption capacity. The fat penetrates the pellets very quickly, before they are hardened. Often the temperatures at the exit of the pellet press, expander or extruder are too high for adding enzymes. Afterwards the pellets are cooled. From a temperature point of view this is a good moment for adding enzymes, but depending on the pellet quality and the design of the cooler there arises an amount of mash that cannot be neglected. This amount of mash has a relatively larger surface than the coarse feed particles and will bind a larger amount of enzyme after spraying. After cooling, however, the mash is sieved and brought back to the pellet press. This is why the enzyme addition needs to take place after the cooling and sieving (Günther and Beudeker, 1997).

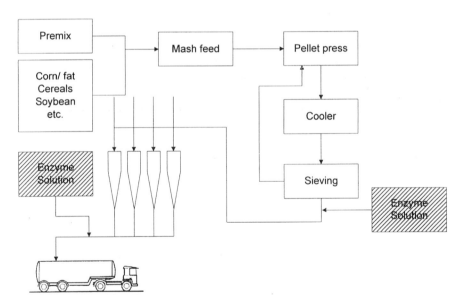

Figure 4.1 Use of liquid heat-sensitive additives, schematic possibilities in the product-line.

Reference: Günther and Beudeker, 1997.

Another possible place for a PPA installation is the bulk loading station. The feed is then sprayed shortly before transporting to the farmer. An advantage of this placing is that only one larger PPA installation is needed per loading station, while placing after the cooler requires a PPA installation for every single press line (Günther and Beudeker, 1997).

Addition of liquid micro-components generally can take place just before or just after coating the feed pellets with fats. Even if the pellets are coated in fat first the low levels of enzyme added can be easily absorbed. The small amount of water added with the enzyme does not alter the humidity of the pellets significantly primarily because addition rates are well below 1 litre/tonne (Perry, 1997). The interaction with fat can also be seen from the research of Annonier et al. (1998), Table 4.1 and Table 4.2.

Table 4.1 Effect of spraying position and time on the recovery of a liquid enzyme.

Diet[a]	Enzyme recovery[b]			
	Control	Enzyme sprayed before fat spraying	Enzyme sprayed immediately after fat spraying	Enzyme sprayed 30 min. after fat spraying
Starter	-	100	90	99
Grower	-	100	104	99

[a]   50% barley based
[b]   2 litres Xylan LC® per tonne of feed
Reference: Annonier et al., 1998.

Table 4.2 Effect of fat level and fat temperature on the recovery of a liquid enzyme.

Fat temperature [°C]	Enzyme recovery [%] in feed with fat level [%][ab]	
	1.5	3.0
64	114	118
80	110	117
88	105	117

[a]   50% barley based
[b]   2 litres Xylan LC® per tonne of feed
Reference: Annonier et al., 1998.

The recovery of Xylan LC® was shown to be sufficient irrespective of the fat temperature or the fat level. Irrespective of the spraying order, feed efficiency was significantly improved by the enzyme in the starting as well as the finishing period: -9 and -4.6% in feed efficiency ratio, respectively (Annonier et al., 1998).

4.1.1   BULK-BLENDING

Changing requirements in the market and limitations imposed during the manufacturing process demand an increased flexibility of outloading systems. One possible solution is to have the variety of products occurring only at the outloading stage (Steen, 1998). In a compound factory equipped with a PPA installation it is possible to produce basic recipes to be stored in the transportation bins. The custom mixes can be made afterwards while loading a lorry or a lorry storage-buffer. In this way there are not so many ready custom mixed storage cells necessary. This is called bulk-blending (De Weert according to Coops, 1997; Van der Steege, 1998; Anonymous, 1998a).

The commonly used traditional production process are usually not flexible enough to meet the market requirements because of the following aspects:
• Allowance needs to be made for special products as early as the dose measurement stages on the milling-mixing line;
• Because specialist additions have to be made as early as the mixing line, there are entrainment problems;
• The effectiveness of certain additives is reduced by heating;
• The size of the production and pelleting runs is determined by small orders;
• The smaller runs account for an inefficient usage of storage capacity.

In the conventional process, all the dose measurement operations are performed in the dose-measurement section, the milling/mixing line or in the pelleting line. In order not to impair the effectiveness of heat sensitive additives, an increasing number of dose measurements are already being carried out during conveyance to the pelleting line. Sometimes the outloading system has facilities for making (manual) additions and for (limited) mixing of products. From figure 4.2 it is clear that a specific customer order has to be tracked by the whole factory (order-oriented production) (Steen, 1998).

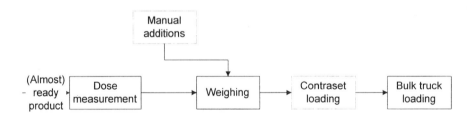

Figure 4.2 Schematic representation of a conventional outloading system.

Reference: Steen, 1998.

To overcome the above-mentioned problems, the specialist additions can be made at the very last moment, just before outloading. This requires expansions at machine level, but it also imposes special demands with regard to operating personnel and to the right automation system (Steen, 1998). Bulk-blending can give the following advantages (Coops, 1997):

- Possibility of blending semi-manufactured feed(compound)s to get the farmer/customer desired composition of the feed. The manufacturer can then produce larger production charges and keep the flexibility in his production line (Heijnen according to Van Vliet, 1998). The changing of products over the pelleting lines will be less as well due to better use of the available finished goods storage (Van der Steege, 1998). A number of semi-finished products can be produced on stock from which the end product is being blended. The costs of raw materials of a blended compound are nevertheless higher than of the same composition, produced in the traditional way. This means that there is a break-even point in the costs. Below a certain order size it is more advantageous to blend; above this size, it is more economical to produce in the traditional way (Van der Steege, 1998).
- Adding of pre-processed raw materials to the finished feed, for example addition of wheat to broiler feed and extra limestone for layers (Van der Steege, 1998).
- Adding of heat sensitive materials without the risk of reducing/destroying the activity of the materials (Heijnen according to Van Vliet, 1998). This can also be done safely in a dosing/coating installation necessary in each pellet line, instead of one system for the central bulk outloading (Van der Steege, 1998).
- Adding of contamination sensitive materials (Van de Weert according to Coops, 1997). Decreasing the contamination in the mill mix process line (Hamers, 1996 and Anonymous, 1997b) and therefore achieving higher hygiene standards (Heijnen, 1998a).
- Adding of fat/oil or sticky materials (Van de Weert according to Coops, 1997).
- Blending and coating to enhance the adhesion of the additives and the wear resistance of the pellet (Steen, 1998).
- Adding of additives in the right dose by dose measurement (Van de Weert according to Coops, 1997).
- Adding of additive to make feed on client specification. These can be liquid or solid additives, from which the concentration differs in the several recipes (Van der Steege, 1998).
- Execution of an extra unit operation, for example crumbling in the bulk outloading (Van de Weert according to Coops, 1997).

Bulk-blending means that the production process is divided into two phases. For an example of fabrication of the basic product and the customised end product, see figure 4.3 (Steen, 1998).

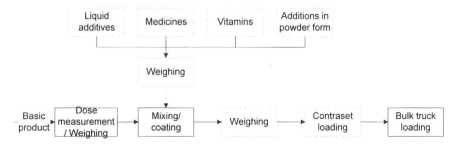

Figure 4.3 Schematic representation of bulk-blending in the outloading.

Reference: Steen, 1998.

A number of possibilities are available to enable bulk-blending during the outloading of finished products. The systems mentioned below all depart from the idea of finished product silos with contra bins or the available height therefore (Van der Steege, 1998).

1. The easiest and most elementary system is that of mixed loading, as seen in figure 4.4. The movable weigher doses the semi-finished products in the contra bins concerned, which similarly unload in the same compartment of the truck. This system is suitable for mixtures of two products in about the same proportion. The accuracy of mixing can not be guaranteed and no liquids can be added. By installing several contra bins on load cells, and equipping them with a dosing element, several semi-finished products can be mixed in different proportions, starting at about 15 percent. The advantage of these systems is that the damage of the product is minimal (Van der Steege, 1998).

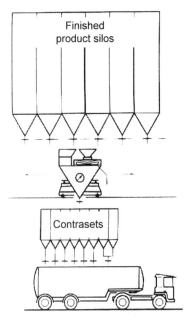

Figure 4.4 Mixed loading, the easiest way of bulk-blending.

Reference: Van der Steege, 1998.

2. The system shown in figure 4.5 is a system in which the blender is mounted beside the contra bins, right under the movable weigher. The weigher receives the different semi-finished products from the finished product silos and discharges them into the mixer. The mixer unloads directly into the truck. The advantage of this system is the limited contamination because of the direct loading. The disadvantage is that no pre-loading is possible, through which the capacity and flexibility are restricted. In the mixer medicines and liquids can be added. The semi-finished products can be sieved in the movable weigher before blending. The installation is relatively simple and suitable when just a small part of the finished product will be blended (Van der Steege, 1998; De Weert according to Coops, 1997).

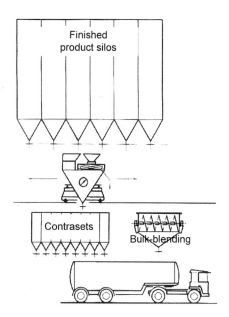

Figure 4.5 Blender besides contra bins.

Reference: Van der Steege, 1998.

3. A development on the above mentioned system is reflected in figure 4.6. Using a transport system, the blended finished product arrives in a little hopper right above the movable weigher. The weigher discharges the product into the contra bin concerned. The flexibility will increase; the capacity however will decrease as the movable weigher will have to transport the product twice. The contamination can be restricted by installing the blender, in which the critical components are being added, above the movable weigher, see right side figure 4.6 (Van der Steege, 1998).

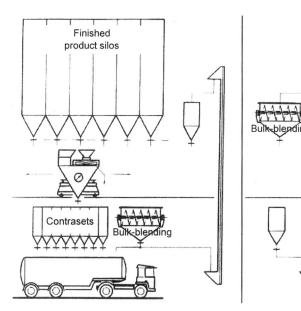

Figure 4.6 Blender in combination with transport system, two different options.

Reference: Van der Steege, 1998.

4. A system, which will not restrict the original loading capacity, is the following. The blender is put on load cells and drives over the same rails as the movable weigher does (see figure 4.7). Both systems can work independently from each other. The control system deals with the priorities, so blender and weigher can not collide. Because of the limited height, the blender is normally not equipped with a sieve. The advantage of this system is the limited contamination because of the separated outloading systems. The complexity of the whole will increase when medicines and liquids are added on the movable blender. The system is suitable for situations in which part of the products will be blended and parts will be delivered directly. When all feed has to pass the blender, the capacity of the blending installation is of great importance (Van der Steege, 1998).

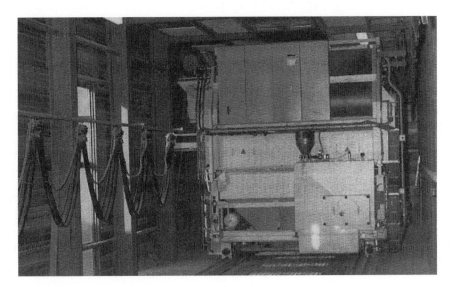

Figure 4.7 Weighing paddle mixer on rails with liquid addition system as installed in a compound feed factory of Gerrits-Jans, Rips, the Netherlands.

Reference: Anonymous, 1997b.

5. To speed up the blending process it can be split up into three sub processes: dosing, mixing and discharge. The capacity of each sub-process can, when critical, determine the overall capacity. An example is shown in figure 4.8. The semi-finished product will be dosed into a weighing hopper through a transport system and a sieve. The mixer will be loaded with pre-weighed components and discharges, after mixing, into a movable under-bin. This will transport the finished product to the contra bins. The capacity of this system is about 60 to 70 tonnes/h. Because all feed will go through the bulk-blending installation, separate enzymes/fat coating installations in the pelleting lines are not required. The installation is also suitable to crumble smaller batches. This can take place independently from the rest of the process. A further increase in capacity (about 70 to 80 tonnes/h) can be achieved by parallel dosing into the mixer and a movable belt to feed contra-bins (Van der Steege, 1998).

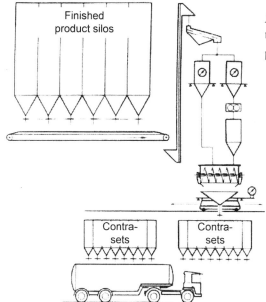

Finished
product silos

Contra-
sets

Contra-
sets

Figure 4.8 Blend installation with movable underhopper.

Reference: Van der Steege, 1998.

If we consider the contamination in more detail, it can be seen that the possibilities for contamination decrease significantly in a bulk-blending system compared to a conventional system, see figure 4.9 (Robohm, 1998). However, the first 4 contamination places shown in the upper figure of 4.9 are nowadays mostly bypassed for additives and premixes: these are added directly to the mixer. According to De Weert (Anonymous, 1998a) the maximum expected contamination or carry-over is 2% against up to 15% in a conventional system (Heeres and Vahl, 1997).

When bulk-blending with a higher capacity is needed, pre-loading in contrasets is preferred, because then the actual loading time of the bulk truck is not affected by the weighing and mixing times (Steen, 1998). With bulk-blending one can anticipate in a very flexible manner, the wishes of the customer (Van der Steege, 1998).

Bulk-blending can be designed in a very flexible way. The danger, in the view of Cebeco Consulting Engineers, is that a complete 'factory' is created after the ready standard product storage. Another disadvantage can be that bulk-blending does not give the opportunity of controlling the end product in time, before it arrives at the customer. Of course samples will be taken and analysed, but the result will often be known when the product is in the silo of the farmer. This is also the case with mixing at the farm, but the latter is the responsibility of the farmer (De Weert according to Coops, 1997).

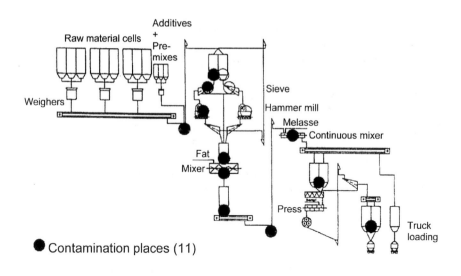

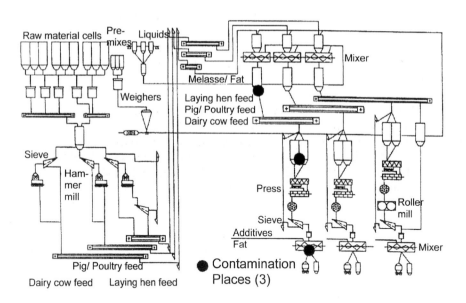

Figure 4.9 Contamination sensitive places in the production line of compound feed, of a conventional feed production line in the upper figure and of a feed production line with bulk-blending in the lower figure.

Reference: Robohm, 1998.

4.2 REQUIREMENTS FOR THE EQUIPMENT

To achieve a homogeneous distribution of additives in feed pellets, the next points can be formulated according to Barendse (1995):
1. The sprayed proportion of feed pellets to the total number of feed pellets needs to be as high as possible.
2. The number of droplets per gram of feed needs to be sufficient.
3. The sprayed pellets need to be mixed as well as possible in the feed, post-mixing.
4. The part of fines and the dust created during or after the post-pelleting application needs to be minimised. Sieving of the fines from the pellets needs to take place before adding the additives.
5. A representative sampling and formulation of the categorised single problems needs to be carried out. This does not influence the homogeneity itself, but is important for analysing the quality of, for example, the homogeneity. This will be discussed in section 5.1.

The number of sprayed pellets in the mixture
A uniform distribution of the additive on the feed pellets is determined by the proportion of sprayed pellets to the total number of pellets to a significant degree. The total installation needs to be designed to reach a coefficient of variation as low as possible. An increasing percentage of sprayed pellets gives the desired decrease in the coefficient of variation. A larger percentage of sprayed pellets can be achieved by special nozzles, see further section 4.3.1, that create a spray curtain, where the pellets are moved through as slowly and turbulently as possible (Günther and Beudeker, 1997).

Even when only 10% of the pellets of a pig feed are sprayed a coefficient of variation of less than 10% can be achieved. Then it is necessary that the sprayed feed particles are distributed homogeneously. In the case of a broiler feed the percentage of sprayed pellets needs to be considerably larger (up to 30%), to reach a coefficient of variation of 10%. The difference is in the smaller number of pellets that a broiler chick consumes daily compared to a finishing pig (200 to 500 pellets per day and 4000 to 20000 per day respectively).

In figure 4.10 a dispersion of additive over feed is shown assuming a Poisson distribution of only 57 droplets per gram of feed, corresponding to a dosage level of 100 ppm and a nozzle generating 150 micron droplets. From this distribution pattern a coefficient of variation of 2.7% can be calculated for samples of 25 grams (Barendse, 1995). In practice the coefficient of variation will be higher since the Poisson distribution assumes that the droplets are dispersed over the feed independently of each other. In reality the droplets are applied to the feed as a mist or curtain of droplets, causing them to behave as if they were less independent droplets.

To approximate a pattern as shown in figure 4.10, the optimal situation, as much as possible; a nozzle type should be chosen with a spraying pattern as wide as possible. In this way the maximum spraying area and therefore maximal dispersion of the liquid spray will be achieved. Additionally, a higher number of droplets per gram could be achieved (Barendse, 1995).

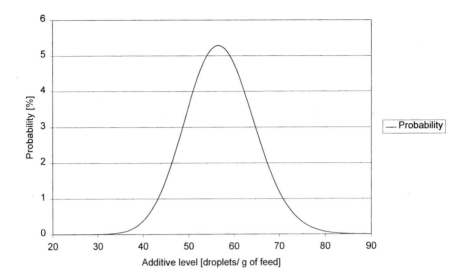

Figure 4.10 Poisson distribution of additive per gram of feed (57 droplets = 100 ppm).

After: Barendse, 1995.

The homogeneous distribution as presented in figure 4.10 seems promising, however it requires more than appropriate spraying equipment to approach it. In practice, it is hardly feasible to disperse the liquid additive over all pellets as is assumed in the equation of figure 4.10. The feed bulk will consist of two fractions; the feed that has been sprayed and the feed that has not been sprayed. Consequently the total variation will consist of at least two contributions as well; the variation due to the distribution of additive over the sprayed feed, more or less according to the description in the preceding paragraph, and the variation caused by the distribution of sprayed pellets over the bulk.

In figure 4.11 the minimal attainable coefficient of variation is depicted as a function of the fraction of feed particles sprayed. In the figure the influence of sample size expressed as number of pellets is also indicated. The sample size can also be read as grams or another weight or volume size. The figure is based on the assumption that all sprayed pellets have the same amount of additive and that sprayed and non-sprayed pellets are mixed completely in the ideal situation. The model-study is made on the assumption of a binomial distribution to take a unit out of a number of units equalling the sample size with the chance equalling the percentage of sprayed pellets to pick a sprayed pellet. From this figure it can be seen that a minimum of 20% of the pellets have to be sprayed if a coefficient of variation of 10% is to be reached in daily ration of chick feed (25 g of 3 mm pellets or 500 pellets). It is also clear that the daily ration of pig feed (1500 g of 5 mm pellets or 6000 pellets) sets much lower demands; only 5% has to be sprayed to reach the same homogeneity (Barendse, 1995 and Günther and Beudeker, 1997). It is clear that much attention has to be paid to the hit level of the feed pellets.

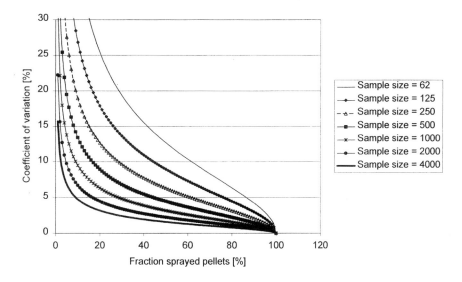

Figure 4.11 Influence of fraction sprayed pellets and sample size (number of pellets or grams) on minimal attainable coefficient of variation in a situation with ideal distribution of the spayed pellets over the total amount of pellets.

After: Barendse, 1995.

Number of droplets
The optimal number of droplets per gram of feed is an arbitration between the desired maximal number of droplets per gram of feed and the maximum amount of liquid, that can be sprayed without decreasing pellet quality. In practice, doses of 0.1 to 0.2% liquid are sprayed on the total feed mixture. At a dose of 0.1% and a given droplet size, about 200 droplets per gram feed are generated. This number is sufficient to reach a homogeneous distribution of the additive in the feed pellets (Günther and Beudeker, 1997).

Mixing
The importance of the mixing step of the sprayed and unsprayed feed pellets in the total PPA process is usually seriously underestimated (Barendse, 1995). Although there is some mixing during transport of the feed, it is expected that the homogeneity will be better, when a complete mixing is performed (Günther and Beudeker, 1997). Figure 4.12 gives an indication of the influence of the mixing process on feed homogeneity. Here, the coefficients of variation of a virtually unmixed and a completely mixed system are given, the last curve corresponding to the data of a 500 pellets/units sample as represented in figure 4.12. Since in practice coefficients of variation of over 100% are impossible it is clear this figure is not completely correct, however, it shows a good argument for mixing (Barendse, 1995).

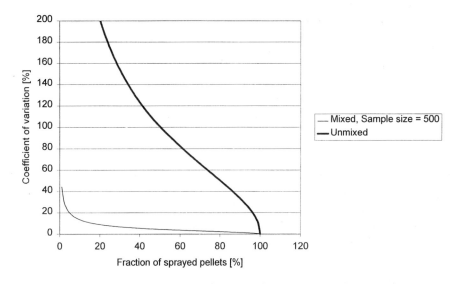

Figure 4.12 Coefficient of variation of unmixed versus well-mixed systems.

Reference: Barendse, 1995.

Segregation and fines

Another important point is the fines, in other words, the segregation of feed particles (Barendse, 1995; Günther and Beudeker, 1997; Van der Poel and Engelen, 1998). It is desirable to sieve the fines before post-pelleting application. Especially in crumb feed, the wide particle size range and the presence of a substantial amount of fines makes the occurrence of segregation practically unavoidable. In pelleted feed care should be taken to minimise the amount of fines. Since the spraying process distributes the liquid components over the available surface, fine particles, having comparatively large surface/weight ratios will absorb a relatively high percentage of the additive. In a feed composed of 95% (by weight) of 3 mm particles with only 5% of 0.5 mm particles the fine fraction can be expected to contain up to 24% of the additive if we assume that the nozzle moistens the surface evenly. (Barendse, 1995; Günther and Beudeker, 1997). If the fines are sieved after spraying of the liquid, considerable amounts of enzymes will be removed out of the feed. Additionally it will cause the bulk of the feed to contain 20% below additive target level (Barendse, 1995).

Segregation is the phenomenon in which mixtures of particles with differing characteristics, separate more or less spontaneously. Segregation due to difference in particle size is probably the widest-known, but segregation can be caused by a host of physical particle characteristics. Differences in size, density, shape, roughness, resilience and aptitude to charge electrically, can lead to difference in particle behaviour when the system is subjected to some source of mechanical agitation (Barendse, 1996).

Fine particles increase the chance of contamination of other batches, especially since the fine particles are apt to spontaneous transport (dusting) and easily remain present in storage and transport equipment (Barendse, 1995). If it is not feasible for the fines to be removed from the feed, substantial improvement might be reached if the PPA system is designed to spray only the coarser fractions on top of an already segregated mixture, or if the fines are made to adhere to the coarser particles, for example, by means of fat addition (Barendse, 1995). The example of severe segregation is also a typical case in which the coefficient of variation loses its original meaning and has only a qualitative value left, since the additive is found in the different samples according to a non-normal distribution (Barendse, 1995).

Attrition of feed pellets after PPA-processing will also generate fine particles, which will have higher additive levels than the bulk. This is caused by the fact that these fines are mainly generated by attrition of the sprayed surface. Although probably lower in additive content than fines already present during spraying, they still present the same risks and care has to be taken when considerable amounts of these fines are found to have formed (Barendse, 1995).

Feed quality in combination with attrition thus has to be a predominant factor in using post-pelleting applications of liquid additives (Van der Poel and Engelen, 1998). In a trial, two diluted additives were sprayed on a pelleted piglet feed, which had an abrasion coefficient of 2.3% fines in the Holmen test. After emptying the spraying unit, the feed was properly sampled. Then, the fines sticking to the wall of the unit were carefully collected for assay, see Table 4.3 (Huber and Gadient, 1998). From this table it is obvious that abraded fines have a ten-fold higher level of liquid additive.

Table 4.3 Recovery of two additives in a pelleted piglet feed and its abraded fines.

Additive	Dose	Found in pelleted feed		Found in fines
		Average [% of total content]	CV [%]	
Vitamin E	50 ppm	73.2	6.6	792 ppm
Phytase	500 U/kg	110.6	15.2	6609 U/kg

Reference: Huber and Gadient, 1998.

Engelen (1998; unpublished data) also studied the effects of attrition and enzyme activity distribution in pellets and fines in post pelleting application of liquid additives in a paddle mixer (Table 4.4).

In this experiment the feed quality has been made worse by adding water. This was done to show the effect of water activity (less important for these results) and decreased feed quality in a paddle mixer. The original (untreated) feed samples showed a Holmen durability of 92.3, a Pfost durability of 98.7 and a Kahl hardness of 10.0 ± 1.7 kg. The feed had a water activity (a_w) of 0.54 and a dry matter content of 897.3 g/kg. In a first preparation after 55 sec mixing while adding 7 litre water to 75 kg feed in a paddle mixer, the samples had the following characteristics: Holmen durability 76.4%, Pfost durability 95.6%, Kahl hardness 2.0 ± 0.5 kg, $a_w = 0.86$ and dry matter content 815.2 g/kg.

Table 4.4 Analysed average xylanase activity of the fraction pellets and fines in 10 samples from a liquid addition experiment with a paddle-mixer.

	Fraction pellets and fines after sieving (3 mm) [%]		xylanase activity in samples [Units/kg]		xylanase activity in one sample (pellets and fines) split up [% activity of samples]		Total xylanase activity in one sample [Units/kg]
	Pellets	Fines	Pellets	Fines	Pellets	Fines	
Average	91.1	8.9	6056	19512	76.4	23.6	7245.5
Standard deviation	2.7	2.7	587.5	216.0	5.8	5.8	747.5
Coefficient of Variation [%]	3.0	30.8	9.7	1.1	7.6	24.5	10.3

Reference: Engelen, 1998; unpublished results.

In a trial 84 ml of xylanase was added to 84 litres of feed (filling level 140%). The total mixing time was 30 seconds, the spraying time 13 seconds after 5 seconds pre-mixing with a conventional nozzle at 3 bar pressure. After the trial samples were taken out of the mixer and separated in a fraction of fines using a 3 mm sieve and a fraction of pellets after spraying of enzyme.

The samples had a reasonably high percentage of fines, this was caused by the addition of water and therefore high water activity. This decreased the hardness and durability of the pellets. The feeds were sieved before delivery by the feed industry. The fines originate from the mixing to add water and the mixing while adding enzyme (Engelen, 1998; unpublished results).

In Table 4.4 is the enzyme activity as analysed for the two separate fractions shown. In this table it is clear that the xylanase activity level of the fines is more than three times higher than the xylanase activity in the pellets. The fines are formed by attrition of the pellets and are therefore from the outer layer of the pellet. It can be concluded from these experiments that the absorption of the enzyme in the pellet is very small, the enzyme is clearly positioned at the outer layer of the pellets (Engelen, 1998; unpublished results).

Other requirements
Enzymes are from a human point of view so-called foreign proteins. These and other additives may cause allergic reactions in sensitive people. Therefore a continued exposure of the personnel to aerosols, for example, does not need to occur. Spray installations need to be placed in closed spray chambers for that reason and the regulations need to be followed (Günther and Beudeker, 1997).

4.3   EQUIPMENT DESIGN

To obtain the desired accuracy and homogeneity, the flow of liquid and feed have to be in close harmony. In principle this can be reached in two ways; either by controlling the feed flow to keep pace with the liquid addition level or vice versa, by controlling the liquid flow to keep it in accordance with the amount of feed passing through the process (Barendse, 1995).

Since the variations normally occurring in feed flow are substantial, for example during the start and end of batch runs, this method sets very high demands on both the liquid spraying system and the control system used. The spraying system should be able to handle a wide range of throughputs, while the response time should be very short to adequately respond to the variations in feed flow. These variations in feed flow combined with the high throughputs make it hardly feasible to rely only on controlling the feed flow, since this will require extensive buffering of the feed. An exception to this condition is the PPA-processing of feed during loading before transport. Here the normal bulk storage silos are used as a buffer, so no additional investments have to be made for intermediate storage capacity (Barendse, 1995).

In practice an economic combination of the two methods is usually employed. This type of system uses limited buffering of the feed flow in combination with a limited variation in liquid addition rate. A typical example is the use of a feed buffer with a high and low indication, from which the feed is drawn at a high rate if the buffer is full and a low rate if the low level is indicated. These high and low rates of feed transports are coupled to the corresponding rates of liquid addition. The extreme case of this method is the batch wise treatment of feed, in which distinct amounts of feed and additive are dosed and mixed. In this case only one liquid dosing rate has to be used, while the capacity of the process has to be sufficiently high to keep ahead of the feed production line (Barendse, 1995).

4.3.1   THE SPRAYING SYSTEM

The spraying process is essentially governed by four parameters (Barendse, 1995), as the current pump technology guarantees that dosing a small amount of 0.002% is no problem:
1. liquid dose level;
2. droplet size;
3. nozzle throughput;
4. spray distribution.

Liquid dose level and droplet size
In figure 4.13 the number of droplets formed per gram of feed is illustrated as a function of the liquid dose level and the droplet size, assuming a bulk density of 1 kg/litre additive. The nozzle throughput usually is fixed by the process capacity and spray or residence time (in batch and continuous processes, respectively) (Barendse, 1995).

It can be seen that much attention has to be paid to the hit level of the feed pellets. A maximisation of the totally sprayed surface by means of one or more wide-angle nozzles is the first step in obtaining a higher fraction of sprayed pellets. A second requisite is the presentation to the spraying process of the maximum number of feed pellets possible by forming a curtain of the feed as wide and turbulently moving as possible. In agitated processes both effects can also be served by prolonging the spraying time when it concerns batch processes and prolonging the feed residence time if continuous processes are concerned (Barendse, 1995).

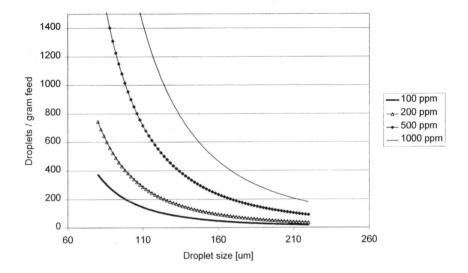

Figure 4.13 Number of droplets formed per gram of feed as a function of the droplet size and additive dosage level, assuming a bulk density of 1 kg/litre additive.

After: Barendse, 1995.

Accurate spray nozzle drop size is an important-factor in the overall effectiveness of a spray operation. To accurately assess drop size for a given nozzle, the evaluation and data collection methods need to be fully understood. The type of instrument, method of collection, manner of interpretation of raw data, and reporting procedures all play a major role in determining drop size performance (Ferrazza et al., 1992).

The American Society for Testing and Materials (ASTM) recognises two different types of drop size sampling techniques; spatial and temporal or flux sensitive. The spatial technique is used when a collection of drops occupying a given volume are sampled instantaneously (see figure 4.14). Generally, spatial measurements are collected with the aid of holographic means or high-speed photography. This type of measurement is sensitive to the number density in each class size and the number of particles per unit volume. The flux-technique is applied when individual drops that pass through the cross section of a sampling region are examined over an interval of time. Flux measurements are generally collected by optical measurements that sense individual drops (Ferrazza et al., 1992).

Flux distribution may be transformed to a spatial distribution by dividing the number of samples in each class size by the average velocity of the drop in that size class. If all drops in a spray are moving at the same velocity, the flux and spatial distribution are identical. However, the spray will generally exhibit differences in drop velocities that vary from class size to class size. In addition these differences depend on the type of nozzle, capacity and spraying pressure (Ferrazza et al., 1992).

* Time averaged
* Sensitive to particle flux

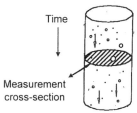

* Averaged over finite volume
* Instantaneous sample
* Sensitive to relative number density N(d), particles/ volume

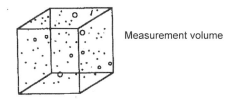

Figure 4.14 The flux measurement in the upper figure versus spatial measurement in the lower figure.

Reference: Ferrazza et al., 1992.

The flux/spatial comparative drop size ratio relationship will vary with pressure. It approaches unity at a condition where all drops would be travelling at the same velocity. Therefore, it is important to combine measurement techniques and equipment for measuring drop diameters. When using the spatial measurement technique, the drop size distribution should be reconciled by applying velocity correction values for each class size in the distribution (Ferrazza et al., 1992).

The Mean Volumetric Droplet diameter (MVD) is in practice often used as a measure of droplet size spectra. Every nozzle creates under a certain spray pressure droplets of differentiating size. Droplet size spectrum means the frequency distribution of the droplet diameter. An MVD of for example 200 µm means, that 50% of the outputted humidity volume is sprayed in droplets with a droplet diameter smaller or equal to 200 µm. Increasing the spray pressure decreases the MVD. The higher the nozzle hole (capacity per time unit), the higher the MVD. In a situation with an equal capacity per time unit and spray pressure, an increasing spray angle decreases the MVD.

From figure 4.13 and Table 4.5 it emerges that large numbers of droplets per gram of feed can be generated by fairly simple equipment even at low dosage levels using undiluted enzyme products (Barendse, 1995). Air assisted nozzles atomise particles, and these are smaller in mass and more numerous than particles from conventional nozzles. In theory, atomisation should provide a more uniform coverage of the feed. However, air currents in feed handling equipment have the potential to blow liquid particles in all directions. Misdirected liquid particles may combine with feed dust and plasticise on surfaces of feed handling equipment. Conventional spray nozzles generate larger liquid droplets that are less affected by air currents in the feed line (Fodge et al., 1997). For addition of molasses and liquid fat, Anonymous (1994a) uses a flat spray nozzle with air atomising, and with air cleaning of the liquid channel after each spray sequence, in order to avoid drops in the mixture. For addition of easy flow, low viscosity liquids, standard one component flat spray nozzles are recommended (Anonymous, 1994a).

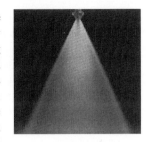

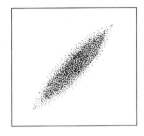

Figure 4.15 Spraying pattern of a flat spray nozzles.

Reference: Anonymous, 1994b.

Table 4.5 General ranges of attainable droplet sizes and number of droplets per millilitre for different nozzle types.

Type nozzle	MVD of spray droplets[a]	Number of droplets per ml
Pneumatic Nozzles	20-400	$2.39*10^5$-29.8
Pressure Nozzles	100-500	$1.91*10^3$-15.3
Rotating Disc Atomisers	20-300	$2.39*10^5$-70.7

[a]   Reference: Barendse, 1995.

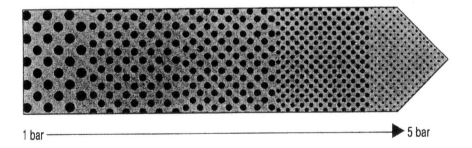

1 bar ⎯⎯⎯⎯⎯⎯⎯⎯⎯⎯⎯⎯⎯⎯⎯⎯⎯⎯▶ 5 bar

Figure 4.16 Droplet size at different pressures for conventional nozzles.

Reference: Anonymous, 1994b.

Micro liquids applicators (Rotating Discs) have some critical design features in common. They eliminate the potential problem of clogged spray nozzles. Instead of using pressurised nozzles, these systems create a fine spray or fog of the liquid by dropping it onto a spinning disk or series of disks. This causes atomisation of the liquid by centrifugal force. The resulting mist permeates a falling curtain or shower of the feed product at or near atmospheric pressure (Abele, 1996).

Nozzle throughput and spray distribution
One factor determining the nozzle throughput and droplet size distribution is the viscosity of the liquid additives or additive mixture (Anonymous, 1998a). Nozzles can only attain a good distribution in a relatively small liquid flow range. When the amounts to spray are too large, then the number of aerosols (creating fog) increases unacceptably. In the case of too small a liquid flow, the spraying cone cannot be maintained, and a homogeneous distribution is not ensured (Günther and Beudeker, 1997). In applications with a continuously changing sort and amount of the additive mixture to be sprayed, it is better to lead every liquid separately from storage to the nozzle (Günther and Beudeker, 1997). In practice pressures of 2 bars and less are most commonly used. When using higher pressures, valves are required close to the nozzle, otherwise the time taken for pressure to build up takes too long (Ouwerkerk, 1997 and Van Leeuwen, 1997).

4.3.2 CONTINUOUS ADDITION OF ADDITIVES

Continuous PPA-installations need to adapt to changes in the product mass flow. For example the pellet press varies considerably in its flow performance within one feed sort. In addition, the used cooling aggregates can bring enormous changes in the mass flow depending on their design. A PPA-installation therefore needs to have an amount registration in the feed route before (Günther and Beudeker, 1997). Also, the on/off timing is very important, the pump must turn on when feed begins flowing past the application site and turn off when feed is not flowing (Fodge et al., 1997).

While this information is known the pump, which pumps the liquid additive or additive mix, must be controlled. In this way, with the change of product mass flow the corresponding additive amount is sprayed. The mass flow registration of pelleted feed is measurable with different kinds of equipment. The next table gives an enumeration of the possible equipment and their accuracy.

Table 4.6 Pellet mass flow-measurement for a continuous working liquid addition system.

Equipment	Accuracy: coefficient of variation [%]
Impact plate weigher	5
Volumetric metering (revolutions controlled feed screw)	5
Feed scroll on balance (running balance)	3
Cell wheel weigher	2
Differential balancing	1

Reference: Günther and Beudeker, 1997.

The necessary space for these measurement systems differs in a widely. While impact plate weighers and cell wheel weighers are very compact equipment, differential weighing requires the most space. Volumetric measurements work only sufficiently accurately when the specific weight of the feed does not differ significantly within a portion of feed, this is only the case when a feed composition and pellet size is as constant as possible. In general, weighing the mass flow is more accurate (Günther and Beudeker, 1997).

The Rotospray of Kahl is used as a continuous liquid additive addition system (Lucht, 1997; Anonymous, 1997d). As mentioned above the product as well as the liquid additives have to be measured, and preferably weighed before they pass the Rotospray (Heijnen, 1998b). Instead of using pressurised nozzles, these systems create a fine spray or mist of the liquid by dropping it without pressure onto a spinning disk or series of disks. This causes atomisation of the liquid by centrifugal force. The resulting mist permeates a falling curtain or shower of the feed product at or near atmospheric pressure (Gill, 1994). Measurements showed that 1 ml liquid is transformed to 10,000,000 droplets (Lucht, 1997). Liquid addition should not exceed 1 to 1.5%, otherwise the advantage of non cross-contamination becomes the disadvantage of product remaining behind causing pollution of all equipment after the Rotospray (Heijnen, 1998b).

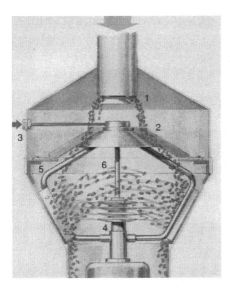

Figure 4.17 The Kahl Rotospray.

1	Material dose system
2	Material curtain (e.g. pellets)
3	Liquid dose system
4	Spinning discs
5	Distribution arm
6	Flow in the spraying chamber

Reference: Anonymous, 1997d.

The system of spraying the additives over the pellets can only be applied to liquids. It is therefore not possible to add powdery additives to the pellets with this system. The maximum percentage of liquids that can be added is limited, due to the continuous dosing process in which the factor time cannot be adjusted. This system can handle up to 5 different liquid micro-ingredients. The maximum capacity of the Rotospray is 120 tons per hour (Heijnen, 1998b).

A similar continuous system was recently launched as the Ring Coater of Schrauwen Trading & Engineering. In this system the pellets fall onto a rotating disc. By centrifugal force the pellets are thrown to the outer wall of the cylinder. The pellets form a curtain that goes down, and the pellets are sprayed with a quick spinning-spraying nozzle. It is possible for three liquids to be dosed and only come together in the nozzle. Company trials showed a good coefficient of variation for a 0.1% dose (Van Laarhoven, 1998).

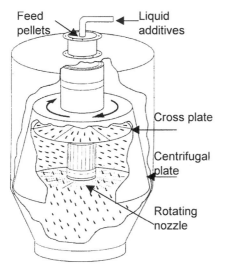

Figure 4.18 The Schrauwen Ring Coater.

Reference: Van Laarhoven, 1998.

Fodge et al. (1997) carried out research in various U.S. feed mills with liquid enzyme addition. A number of mills with roto-coaters were examined. A roto-coater is a barrel-shaped apparatus with a rotating, hollow drive shaft through its centre. The pelleted feed enters the roto-coater through an inlet chute at the top and drops onto the feed handling disc, which rotates at a slow to moderate speed. The rotation of the feed handling disc uniformly throws the feed against the cylindrical walls of the coater and the feed then falls past the liquid disc, which is positioned in the centre of the cylindrical flow of feed. Normally fat is coated with this disc. It is however possible to also spray enzymes simultaneously with the fat. In figure 4.19 some of the results from different mills and feed lines are presented.

Both the systems F and G are continuously fed systems in which an impact-style load cell is positioned in the feed line just prior to the roto-coaters. Feed strikes the impact plate, and a proportional voltage signal from the feed line just prior to the roto-coaters. As feed strikes the impact plate, a signal from the impact plate is forwarded to a control for the output of the fat and the enzyme pumps in synchrony with the feed flowing into the roto-coaters. Feed slides off the impact plate in a curtain-shape, roughly 5 cm thick and 40 cm wide, directly above the roto-coater. One spray nozzle is positioned on either side of this curtain and sprays the enzyme on the feed, rather than applying it inside the roto-coater (Fodge et al., 1997).

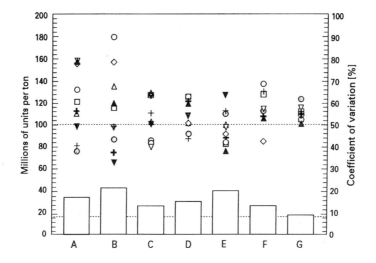

Figure 4.19 Application of roto-coaters for adding liquid enzymes.

- Lower dotted line is the CV obtained from spraying the enzyme in a batch mixer.
- Upper dotted line is the desired amount of enzyme per ton applied to the feed.
- Above each letter are 10 data points where each point represents the average enzyme activity for 10 sets of 10 feed samples (one set collected in about 60 seconds) over several weeks.

Reference: Fodge et al., 1997.

In the upper figure of 4.20 the data collected from four feed lines where the enzyme was applied by spraying it on curtains of feed falling from the end of weigh-belt coaters are shown. Spray nozzles for spraying fat have been positioned on either side of this curtain. For adding enzyme nozzles have been positioned on both sides of the curtain of feed, either above or below the fat nozzles and occasionally, have included the enzyme with the fat (Fodge et al., 1997).

Several other sides have been examined by Fodge et al. (1997). The lower figure of 4.20 shows systems A, B, C and D that represent attempts to spray the enzyme on the feed as it falls from the end of a cooler belt, at the load-out chute above the trucks, and two sides beneath the canopy of the two separate pellet dies, as the feed falls from the pellet die into the cooler. Neither the CVs (all > 30%) nor the accuracy of these applications were acceptable. Feed falling off a cooler belt is often too thin a curtain and the sprayed solution penetrates the curtain resulting in a liquid build-up on the surfaces of the production equipment. At load-out, the chute dropping feed into the truck bins was equipped with a nozzle on each side, but the feed falls too fast and thickly. Neither of the pellet mill canopy applications worked well because of fluctuating air current, and the hot feed decreasing the yield of product (Fodge et al., 1997).

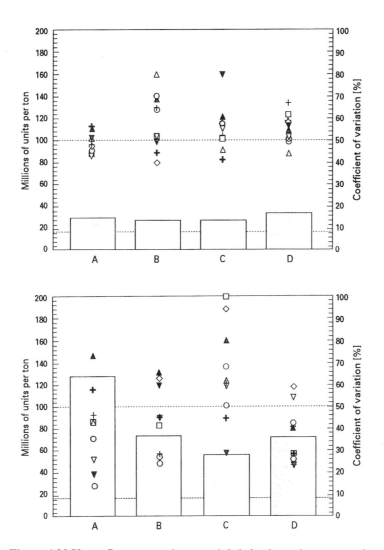

*Figure 4.20 Upper figure: spraying at weigh-belts through spray nozzles,
A = constant rate, B-D = varying rate.*

*Lower figure: Spraying at various sides A-load out, B-cooler, C & D-under pellet
mill.*

- Lower dotted line is the CV obtained from spraying the enzyme in a batch mixer.
- Upper dotted line is the desired amount of enzyme per ton applied to the feed.
- Above each letter are 10 data points where each point represents the average enzyme
  activity for 10 sets of 10 feed samples (one set collected in about 60 seconds) over
  several weeks.

Reference: Fodge et al., 1997.

4.3.3 DISCONTINUOUS ADDITION OF ADDITIVES

Discontinuous working, batch type PPA-installations are not dependent on changes in the product mass flow. These installations are built up with a spray chamber, often in the form of a quickly rotating mixer. The mixer is placed on a balance, the amount of feed to spray is weighed immediately in this case. Usually the same amount of pellets will be sprayed, and the same amount of enzyme or enzyme mix will have to be sprayed (Günther and Beudeker, 1997).

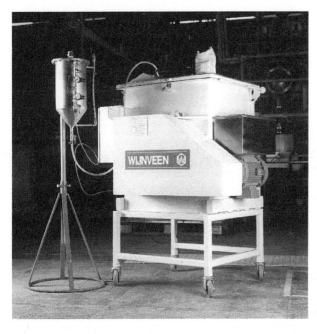

Figure 4.21 F-60 discontinuous paddle mixer with liquid addition system pressure drum, used as a demonstration model.

In this way the mixer can form a bulk-blending unit in addition to liquid addition (section 4.1.1). In mixing, a lot of problems can exist. Often the importance of mixing, as mentioned earlier, is underestimated. Often, the mixer is the bottleneck in the production process (Røsjorde, 1992). Problems occurring in mixing and mixers are (Røsjorde, 1992):

- Poor mixing quality can create pockets of unmixed material in the mixer;
- It is difficult or impossible to add liquid, because the liquid and product can stick to the mixing tools in such a way, that the mixing ability is greatly hampered;
- Sensitive for over- and under filling;
- Long mixing time can in many cases reduce the quality of the product, and overformulating may be necessary to compensate;
- Emptying often takes place through a small hole in the bottom of the mixer, which creates a tremendous segregation during discharging;
- The mixer needs to be large to have enough capacity, thus creating the need for large hoppers above and below the mixer, so the space requirement can be vast.

In mixers with a normal filling level coefficients of 3-4% are possible. For charges of 40-50% of the designed filling level of a mixer, the coefficient of variation increases to 10-11% (Heeres and Vahl, 1997).

Theoretically three different types of mixtures distinguished: ideal, random and ordered mixtures (Barendse, 1996; Røsjorde, 1992). Each one will be explained in the following paragraphs.

Ideal mixture

Maybe the ideal mixture in figure 4.22 (left) is readily recognised as a homogeneous mixture but it is never encountered in reality. The truly ideal symmetrical distribution of the different particles characteristic for this type of mixture is never accomplished by a realistic mixing process (Barendse, 1996; Røsjorde, 1992).

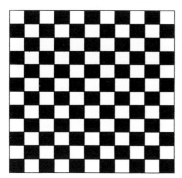
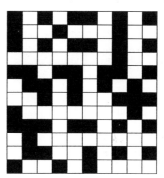

Figure 4.22 Left: Completely ordered distribution of particles, the Chess board pattern. Right: Random distribution of particles.

Reference: Barendse, 1996; Røsjorde, 1992.

Random mixture

In comparison, the random mixture, see figure 4.22 (right), appears less homogeneous, mainly because of its lack of symmetry. Despite this outward appearance we will see later that when such a mixture is judged on its homogeneity on a realistic scale, it will prove virtually as homogeneous as the ideal mixture. The ideal random mixture is only approximated in real mixing. During the mixing process the separation in the mixture existing at the start will be diminished progressively in time, and even in the absence of segregation, the ideal random state is never completely reached. As in diffusion processes the driving force for the mixing phenomenon (diminishing differences) is reduced as the mixing progresses, thereby reducing the effectiveness of further mixing. Mixing progress can therefore often be described according to some first order function. A realistic mixture that is achieved during mixing processes will usually show a random distribution of clusters of particles. During the mixing process these clusters will become progressively smaller eventually approaching the scale of the individual particles, thus approaching an ideal random mixture (Barendse, 1996).

Ordered mixture

The ordered mixture is a special case, the different particle species are not randomly mixed but ordered, thus looking more like an ideal mixture. Such an ordered mixture may result from blending of a fine, cohesive powder with a coarser one. In this case, the fine powder particles may distribute over and adhere to the surface of the coarser material. When sampled, this mixture may be found to be more homogeneous than expected based on calculations assuming random mixture (Barendse, 1996).

Levy-flight

There is a theory in mixing called 'Levy flight', see figure 4.23. This mixing process consists of convection and diffusion. It consists of relatively long movement of the particles, whereas the particles get very intimately mixed. Then new long movements of particles occur and so forth. Without the convection part of the mixing, it will only be diffusion, and it will take an extremely long time before the mixture is homogenised. On the other hand, if we are going to rely only on convection, it also takes a much longer time until the mixture is homogenised, because we have to cut through the mixture and move particles all the time. In practice it will take too much time until the mixer has cut through the smallest segment of the mixture. If a mixer combines both convection and diffusion, the mixture can be achieved in reasonable time. If these principles are combined, the mixer can mix under weightless conditions, so there will be no segregation of ready mixed material. The mixture can then be ready in a short period of time with an unknown degree of precision (Røsjorde, 1992).

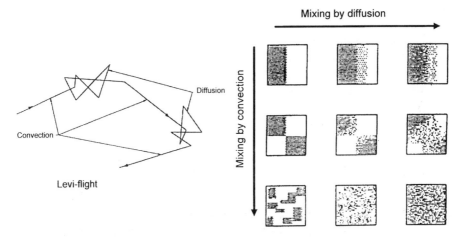

Figure 4.23 Schematic representation of one particle in levy flight, left and a schematic representation of convection and diffusion mixing, right.

Reference: Røsjorde, 1992.

The paddle mixer can be used for premix and concentrate production, for compound feed production, for additive addition just before the bulk-outload and for blending half-fabricates or end-products in the bulk-outload section as a stationary mixer or as a mixing bulk-robot (Heijnen, 1998b). There are several compound feed machine builders producing paddle mixers, with two rotors.

In a paddle mixer, the rotors overlap in the centre of the mixer, and the paddles completely sweep the bottom, and mix all the material at the same time. When we look at one rotor, each round of paddles is formed by three paddles to one side and one paddle to the other side, in each quadrant of the drum. When the paddles of one rotor rotate they pick the material between the paddles of the other rotor up. There will be a circulating material stream in zone 'B', the bottom layer of the mixer, while in zone 'A', above the material surface mechanical fluidisation is achieved, in which the particles are randomly scattered around (single particle Levy flights)

(Van Aken, 1996). It is important that the zone of mixing, in the centre between the paddle shafts, is large enough that there is enough diffusion to perfect the mixing. In the centre between the shafts, there is about 60% of the material mechanically fluidised. This means the material is not exposed to the segregation caused by gravity. All the used energy can be applied for creating the perfect mixture in this case while no energy is needed for recreating the mixture being segregated during the mixing process (Røsjorde, 1992).

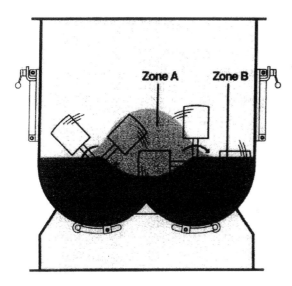

Figure 4.24 The different mixing zones in a paddle mixer.

Reference: Anonymous, 1994b.

To increase the capacity of these discontinuous working PPA-installations, the spray chamber mixer needs a buffer storage in front and at the end. In this way the mixer can be loaded and unloaded at once. The total time for loading, spraying, homogenising and unloading can be done in less than 60 seconds in this way. A mixer with 250 kg volume is sufficient for a pellet line with a capacity of 10-15 ton/h (Günther and Beudeker, 1997).

Optimal contact between the droplets of a nozzle and the feed particles can be achieved by increased free surface of the pellets. This can be done by creating free space between the particles. This goal is reached by forcing the particles with a movement in a fluidisation zone or a free fall (Van der Poel, 1996). The liquid will be added by a nozzle mounted in the lid pointed towards the outer rim of the fluidised zone (zone 'A') of the mixer (Anonymous, 1994b).

Liquid dosing in a paddle mixer is possible in several ways, as shown in figure 4.25. When using a flow distortion bar (FDB) during spraying into powders, the liquid shall be sprayed into the curtain of material. When coating fragile materials like pellets, cereals, etc., FDB must not be used. The mixer must be overfilled by 20-40% when using the FDB (Anonymous, 1994b).

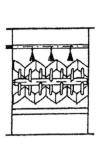

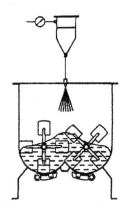

Liquid addition direcly by holed pipe into the centre of the mixer

Liquid addition trhough flat spray nozzle into the fluidized zone

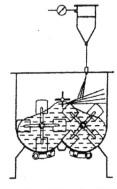

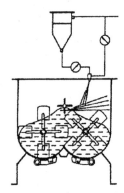

Liquid addition by FDB and flat spray nozzle

Liquid addition by FDB and flat spray nozzle with air atomizing

Figure 4.25 Possibilities for liquid dosing in a paddle mixer.

Reference: Anonymous, 1994b.

The following parameters are decisive for choosing the method:
- The particles' shape;
- The particles' size;
- Hygroscopic characteristics;
- Amount of liquid to be added;
- The liquid viscosity;
- Homogeneity;
- Accuracy.

Positioning of the nozzles in the lid of paddle mixers is in practice a problem. In the lid there must be a main filling hole and often more filling holes for adding solid by-components. Therefore the area for placing nozzles is limited and is often not ideal.

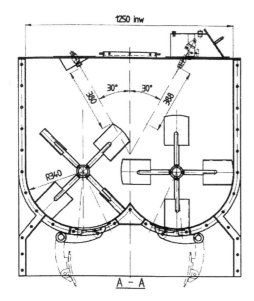

Figure 4.26 Upper figure: Positioning of nozzles from a cross-sectional viewpoint in a paddle mixer. The two nozzles require different heights and have different closing systems, one is closed by a needle, the other by valves before the nozzle. Each requiring his own build in position and method.

Lower figure: Schematic top view of a paddle mixer, Wijnveen-Forberg F350 with positioning of spraying equipment, fat spraying and phytase spraying.

Reference: Anonymous, 1997c.

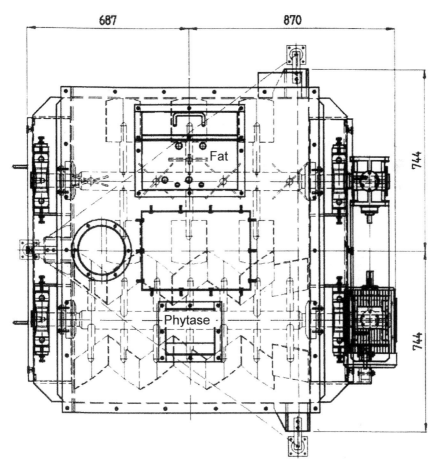

In figure 4.26 a practical example is viewed. In this mixer, an F-350, a phytase and a fat spraying nozzle had to be placed as well as the main filling hole and an extra grain-filling hole. Therefore the positions of the nozzles are pushed more to the sidewalls.

The nozzles are preferably not placed too close to the holes in case of repairs and dust build up on the nozzles when dust is formed during filling of the mixer. The nozzle can thus not be placed directly above the fluidised zone, so they have to spray from an angle in the fluidised zone. The nozzles then have to be positioned under an angle in the lid and moreover have to be placed in a way reachable for adjustment of position, cleaning and repairing. The same mixer is also shown in figure 5.3 in cross-section. In this figure it is clear that different nozzles have different requirements for mounting and positioning.

According to the producers of the Wijnveen-Forberg mixers, these mixers are able to *mix* satisfactorily at filling levels between 40 and 140% of the normal content (Anonymous, 1997c), see figure 4.27. For adding liquid it is recommended to use a higher filling level than 100% to increase the recovery. At 100% filling level the amount of liquid sprayed directly on the paddles is too high, a filling level of 140% is recommended.

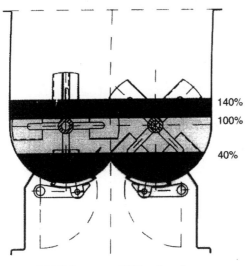

Figure 4.27 Filling levels of the Forberg mixer.

Reference: Anonymous, 1994b.

140%
100%

40%

100% is normal filling level.

4.3.4   BATCH SYSTEM VERSUS CONTINUOUS SYSTEM

A continuous liquid adding type requires extra accuracy in determining the pellet flow and the liquid flow. Quick control and steering of the liquid flow is important with a variable pellet flow. In absence of pellets, the liquid flow needs to stop immediately. It is even better not to spray beneath a certain pellet flow because in low flows the pellet-curtain is not closed. In a batch system the exact amount of pellets is known and the exact amount of liquid can be balanced. In this system there is accordingly no need for continuous control of the liquid flow (Nijskens, 1993). From an investment-cost point of view a batch system is cheaper because there can be savings on a mass registration system (Günther and Beudeker, 1997).

When the desired amount is reached, the additive is sprayed within 20-30 seconds in the quick rotating mixers (Günther and Beudeker, 1997). Using buffer storage in before and after the mixer, a capacity of ± 90 tons per hour is possible (Van der Steege, 1998). A continuous system can reach a flow of ± 90 tons per hour (Heijnen, 1998b)

In trials in England (Nijskens, 1993), batch systems have proved to be more accurate than continuous systems, mainly implied by the ease of measuring and controlling pellet and liquid flows. Another advantage of the paddle mixers is that not only liquids but also powders can be added to the product (Heijnen, 1998b). Therefore this type of mixer gives the possibility of bulk-blending.

5 ANALYSING FEED QUALITY

5.1 SAMPLING

It is important to measure differences in the amount of additives at several positions in the mixer after the mixing process. To determine the distribution of additives after spraying, we need to set up a standard procedure for taking the samples in the mixer.

Sample size
A sample should always contain so many particles (n) that the coefficient of variation will be considerably smaller than the minimal value that should still be detectable. Often the most realistic sample size is dictated by the application. If the coefficient of variation is still too high in this case, there remains no other option than to mill the particles down to a smaller size and thus increase the number of particles (n) (Barendse, 1996). In the feed industry often a sample size is taken as big as a day ration of the animal the feed will be applied to (Barendse, 1995). In figure 5.1 it is clear that if the sample size increases by a factor of 5 the measured coefficient of variation will be half of the original value (Barendse and Van Doesum, 1993). The effect of the sample size was modelled by a binomial distribution.

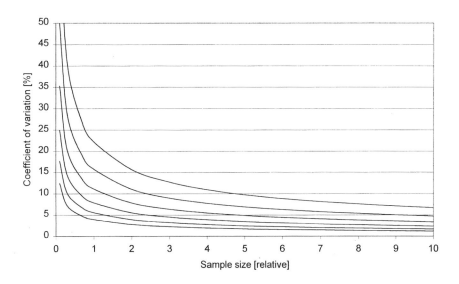

Figure 5.1 Relative influence of sample size on coefficient of variation.

Reference: Barendse, 1995.

Number of samples
A realistic number of samples is often more difficult to decide on, since the accuracy of the estimation of the coefficient of variation will increase with the number of samples, but so will the analysis costs. The required accuracy and associated cost will have to be balanced against each other for each case separately. In production situations, numbers of samples can be kept relatively limited when evaluation data on subsequent batches can be put together to give an overall distribution performance with increasing accuracy (Barendse, 1996).

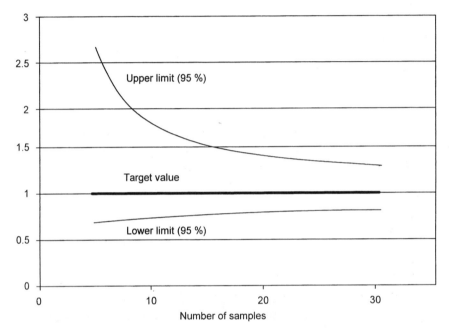

Figure 5.2 Confidentially interval for calculated standard deviation.

Reference: Barendse, 1995.

It is important to take representative samples of the involved batch of feed, particularly if the particle size distribution of the feed is wide. This can lead to separation, which complicates taking representative samples (Barendse and Van Doesum, 1993).

In a batch mixer it is important to take the samples in the mixer and not after unloading, because unloading effects the uniformity of the batch of feed. To sample within the mixer one has to have a device to take samples in the bottom as well as the top layer of feed without disturbing or mixing the feed. In practice this is not possible, but disturbing has to be minimised. In unpublished experiments (Engelen, 1998) a special sample device was developed for this purpose. The enclosed device, shown in figure 5.3 was pushed into the feed while the feed was still in the mixer, the device was opened and collected the sample which fell into the cylinder, enclosed the sample in the cylinder and was pulled out of the feed again. The sample device was manoeuvred between the paddles to collect the samples from the bottom layer. A fixed sample size and sampling procedure is recommended, however this can involve practical problems.

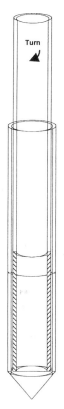

5.2 TRACERS

The measurement of the dose accuracy can be done with the additive itself or a tracer that is not used in normal feeds. In this case the known amount of tracer is dissolved in a known amount of liquid additive. Samples of the marked additive and the unsprayed feed can be taken as blanks. After spraying we can take samples and perform chemical analyses to calculate recovery and coefficient of variation (Van der Poel, 1996). Cobaltchloride (Heeres and Vahl, 1997) or vitamin C-derivatives are appropriate tracers (Nijskens, 1993). In unpublished experiments (Engelen, 1998), Cobalt Ethylene Di Tetra Acetic acid (EDTA) was used as a tracer. This is another derivative of Cobalt, and as with Cobaltchloride the concentration of Cobalt is determined after the experiment. Cobalt EDTA is used in animal nutrition exclusively as a tracer and has no nutritional value. Normally feeds do not contain Cobalt in the recipe.

Figure 5.3
Sample
device.

The analysis of the added tracer Co EDTA can be done in a similar way to NEN 3349. In this analysis 5 grams of the feed sample with the added tracer is weighed. This feed was burned in the oven to destroy all organic bondings. Afterwards the sample is cooked dry in a HCl solution (10 ml), dissolved in HCl again (5 ml) and then diluted with water to 50 ml. Of these 50 ml a sample can be taken to analyse using the spectra analyser at 270.7 nm (± 0.2 nm). According to the used manual, NEN 3349, the duplo analysis has to be within 15% of the average of the sample analysed in twofold. In practice the duplos were mostly within 5% of the average. This analysis is relatively simple and inexpensive (Coolen, 1998).

6 CONCLUSIONS AND RECOMMENDATIONS

6.1 CONCLUSIONS

Liquid addition of feed additives may give a solution in many cases to making the ready product assortment more flexible. This will cause an extra capital investment that can be earned back by better efficiency and a larger product assortment (Coops, 1997).

In practice a rule of thumb states that when processing temperatures exceed 75 °C, enzymes should be added after the heat treatment (Günther and Beudeker, 1997). Mixtures of liquid additives are not always possible. Liquid additive mixtures have to be examined for their physical-chemical compatibility before being used. Enzymes to be used simultaneously, should, if possible, be treated and dosed separately (Günther and Beudeker, 1997). For quality application it is necessary to take the analyses and labelling according to the government into account (Coops, 1997).

There are possibilities for continuous as well as discontinuous post-pelleting applications. Discontinuous apparatus are easier to control and adjust. Discontinuous systems have the advantage that no on-line mass flow determination of additive and feed is required; however continuous systems are often more compact (Günther and Beudeker, 1997). In terms of quality, the literature shows that using a batch paddle mixer in a bulk-blending application contamination hardly occurs (0.5%) in a full mixer without liquid addition. This will be higher at a filling level of 40% or less, in which case product can stay on the axes (Coops, 1997).

In a post-pelleting application with bulk-blending one can anticipate in a very flexible manner the wishes of the customer. The possibilities for the application of bulk-blending are various (Van der Steege, 1998):
- Semi-finished products;
- Raw materials;
- Fat coating;
- Additives (dry or liquid).

In practice it is generally agreed that the accuracy of spraying liquid additives, measured by coefficients of variation should be within 10% (Beumer, 1991; Wicker and Poole, 1991; Barendse, 1993; Günther and Beudeker, 1997; Heidenreich, 1998) with a sample size as big as the daily ration of the animal. This means a less critical distribution for animals with a higher feed consumption. This value includes variation from sampling procedure, assay method, randomness, and mix uniformity (McCoy et al., 1994). For mutual additives the effects of a varying coefficient of variation will be different and possibly different goals have to be defined. McCoy et al. (1994) concluded out of a mixing uniformity experiment with broiler chicks that depending on the uniformity test used, CV of up to 20% may be adequate for maximum growth performance. This would give a new point of view on the implications of adding liquid additives and needs further examination. According to Schwarz (1998b) a variation coefficient of less than 20% for phytase should be sufficient.

The analysis accuracy plays an important role in the overall accuracy determined for the liquid addition. If the analysis of the pure additive and the feed have an equal relative accuracy, it is difficult to give reliable estimations in terms of recovery. If dosing for example 0.1% with an analysis accuracy of 5%, the maximal deviation of the analysis is 50 times the dose. Therefore the use of tracers with a high analysis accuracy and the development of measurement techniques with a higher accuracy can contribute to a better determination of the distribution of additives in feed. In unpublished measurements (Engelen, 1998) with Cobalt Ethylene Di Tetra Acetic acid (EDTA), according to the used manual, NEN 3349, the duplo analysis of Co EDTA has to be within 15% of the average of the sample analysed in twofold. Co EDTA analysis, however can have an accuracy of ± 5% in feed (Coolen, 1998). At the moment Co EDTA is a good tracer to use for uniformity experiments, if the accuracy of ± 5% in feed (Coolen, 1998) can be achieved. The analysis of Co EDTA is relatively easy and not costly. It is however, preferable to be able to determine a tracer in feed with more accuracy. This is possible improving the analysis method or using new tracers. A higher accuracy would allow much better recovery calculations when the analysis fault on the pure additive can be much less than the dosing level.

It can be concluded that the positioning of the nozzle is very critical. The spraying cone projection (area) on the feed has to be maximised without spraying directly on the sidewalls. Therefore the spraying cone has to be projected only at the fluidised zone. For the design this means that a nozzle with a very small oval projection parallel to the axes of the paddles in the fluidised zone not quite reaching the side walls will be the best, as shown in figure 6.1. In the fluidised zone the free area of the pellets is as large as possible, the hit rate will then be the highest. When using a nozzle with a wide spray pattern, close to the sidewalls, one has to be careful with the filling level. Too low a filling level will cause the nozzle to spray directly on the sidewalls. More research on recovery will also have to be done to make a definite conclusion about the best filling level. For investing in a paddle mixer for liquid addition one of the main considerations determining the size of the mixer has to be the possibility of using the best filling level as many times as possible.

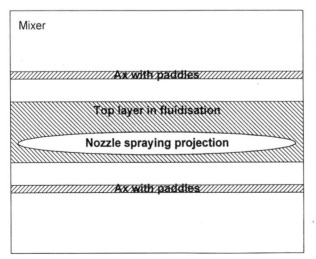

Figure 6.1 Best spraying area in a paddle mixer.

The sample size is critical in the judgement of coefficients of variation as a means of evaluating distribution. When considering a sample size as big as the daily ration of an animal, a chick has a daily ration of 25 g while a sow has a minimum daily ration of 1500 g. In literature there are no clear recommendations for the sample size in accordance with a judgement of the coefficient of variance. This judgement is individually different and dependant on other parameters (such as type of additive, animal concerned etc.). Recommended is a fixed sample size and sampling procedure, this can however, involve practical problems. Introducing a standard sample size all over the world for these kind of experiments should be considered to increase the comparability of experiments all over the world.

Out of the literature review the following points can be formulated for research and application of post-pelleting processes:
- Maximisation of the sprayed fraction of feed;
- Distribution and droplet size of the liquid spray;
- Thorough mixing of the sprayed feed;
- Presence or formation of fines during and after PPA-processing;
- Precise equipment;
- Stability and loss of active substances/carry-over;
- Evaluation procedure of determining homogeneity, in sampling and analysing.

It seems that a coefficient of variation of 10%, which is generally accepted in industry (Beumer, 1991; Wicker and Poole, 1991; Barendse, 1993; Günther and Beudeker, 1997; Heidenreich, 1998), is hard to reach under critical circumstances (Engelen, 1998; unpublished data). Besides that, in an experiment (Engelen, 1998; unpublished data) it was shown that the fines in the pellets had a more than three times higher additive content than the pellets (19512 ± 216 versus 6056 ± 587 Units/kg enzyme). Therefore the industry has to be cautious with the implementation of post-pelleting applications. The choice between dry or liquid addition of feed additives is not as simple as price or convenience although they have a major impact (Blair, 1996). The quality of liquid addition has an impact on feed intake as well as on animal performance. These items in particular have to be examined in relation to different types of feed additives. Further investigations regarding the uniformity, contamination and separation are important to determine the field of application (Van der Steege, 1998). This research is important for the animal feed manufacturer for whom the application of liquid additives will be an indispensable tool for flexible and accurate production (Van der Poel and Engelen, 1998).

6.2 RECOMMENDATIONS

From the unpublished experiments (Engelen, 1998), section 4.2, it is clear that the xylanase activity level of the fines is more than three times higher than the xylanase activity in the pellets. It can be concluded from these experiments that the absorption of the enzyme in the pellet is very small, the enzyme actually stays on the outer layer of the pellet. The fines are formed by attrition of the pellets and originate therefore from the outer layer of the pellet, causing them to have a high activity level. Probably in an application where vacuum is used while spraying additives, it may be possible to achieve absorption of the additives more properly (deeper) into the pellets. The problem of attrition after and during mixing can then be reduced. Further research should be carried out to examine the possibilities of spraying under vacuum. In addition, research should be done to decrease the mechanical stress in feed handling equipment so less fines are formed. This must be combined with improving the feed quality in terms of pellet durability and hardness.

With respect to the positioning of the additive in or on the pellet and feed quality, the absorption capacity of different pellets with the use of different liquids has to be examined/studied.

Not all additives are presently available in a fluid form as a suspension or an emulsion. About the compliance with other additives there has been until now little information known (Wagner, 1998). Further investigations in mixing liquids, stability of liquid formulated additives and the relationship between the viscosity and other liquid properties on the droplet size and droplet distribution of a nozzle have to be done.

It would be of great interest to show the effects of distribution of a liquid additive for example an enzyme on an animal feed to the performance and health status of an animal. To get a critical experiment, a sensitive animal with a low feed consumption per day can be used, for example laying hens, broilers or piglets. For example McCoy et al. (1994) concluded from a mixing uniformity experiment with broiler chicks that depending on the uniformity test used, CV of up to 20% may be adequate for maximum growth performance in broiler chicks. This might lead to a reconsideration of the generally accepted uniformity level of the industry (< 10%). This can give a new point of view on the implication of adding liquid additives.

Cost analysis, between the traditional compound manufacturing process and the addition of liquid additives after pelleting in a bulk-blending process line can give a better insight into the economic possibilities. The capacity and flexibility of the production line should be taken into account.

Further research on the recovery as well as the distribution in a paddle mixer with varying filling levels has to determine the best filling level for a paddle mixer as a percentage of the normal filling level.

For addition of liquid additives in a paddle mixer the following parameters have to be analysed in uniformity and recovery:

1. Concerning the equipment
   - Varying mixing time, especially post spraying time;
   - Filling level;
   - Varying spraying time;
   - Varying different types of nozzles, pressurised and conventional;
   - Varying pressure;
   - Varying spraying position;
   - Varying width of spraying projection of the nozzle;

2. Concerning feed
   - Adding fat simultaneously, before or after adding liquid additives;
   - Porosity of pellets versus absorption of additives;
   - Feed quality of pellets;
   - Particle size and particle size distribution.

REFERENCES

Abele U.; 1996; *A new production method of feed containing pharmacologically active substances by spraying on micro liquids downstream from pelleting, expansion and extrusion*; Internal report Chevita GmbH; Pfaffenhofen, Germany; 8 p.

Albers, N.; 1996; *The influence of the production process and the composition of the mixture on vitamin stability*; Feed Compounder; Nr. April; p. 12-14.

Annonier, C., P.A. Geraert, A. Sabatier and T. Julia; 1998; Proceedings 4th Kahl Symposium; Hamburg, Germany.

Anonymous; 1994a; *Forberg Machinery, mixing – cooling – drying – granulating*; Halvor Forberg A/S; Larvik, Norway; Product information.

Anonymous; 1994b; *Industriële Sproeiers*; Spraying Sytems Nederland B.V.; Schiedam, The Netherlands; Product information.

Anonymous; 1997a; *Study guide "Applicaties van kwaliteitszorg in de dierlijke productie" E200-209*; Sub departments Veehouderij, Veefokkerij, Veevoeding en Levensmiddelentechnologie; Wageningen, The Netherlands; 10 p.

Anonymous; 1997b; *Schonere productie*; Voerpers; Gerrits-Jans Veevoederfabrieken b.v.; Bakel, The Netherlands; Nr. 10; p. 7.

Anonymous; 1997c; *De Wijnveen "Forberg" menger*; Wijnveen Ede b.v.; Ede, The Netherlands; Product information.

Anonymous; 1997d; *Sprühsystem für flüssige Zusatzstoffe: Rotospray®*; Amandus Kahl; Hamburg, Germany; Product information.

Anonymous; 1998a; *IFF-Kolloquium '98:"Flexibilität im Mischfutterwerk"*; Die Mühle + Mischfuttertechnik; Vol. 135; Nr. 22; p. 752-754.

Anonymous; 1998b; *Nordische EU-Länder: Fütterungsantibiotika*; Die Mühle + Mischfuttertechnik; Vol. 135; Nr. 24; p. 818.

Barendse, R.C.M.; 1993; *De verwerking van Natuphos: zowel droog als vloeibaar; Mestprobleem of menuprobleem?: Presentation 2nd Phytase day, 11 February 1993*; Gist-brocades; Rijswijk, The Netherlands; p. 1-11.

Barendse, R.C.M. and J.H. van Doesum; 1993; *Toepassing van vloeibare veevoederenzymen na het pelleteren*; de Molenaar; Vol. 96; Nr. 51/52; p. 1471-1477.

Barendse, R.C.M.; 1995; *Technological Aspects of Enzyme Usage*; Victam '95, Symposium: From Feed to Food; Utrecht, The Netherlands; 11 p.

Barendse, R.C.M.; 1996; *PAON cursus mengen en agglomereren: Mixing and Segregation of Particulate Systems*; Putten, The Netherlands; 15 p.

Bedford, M.R. and Classen, H.L.; 1992; *Reduction of intestinal viscosity through manipulation of dietary rye and pentosanase concentration is effected through changes in the carbohydrate composition of the intestinal aqueous phase and results in improved growth rate and food conversion efficiency in broiler chicks*; Journal of Nutrition; Vol. 122; p. 560-569.

Beumer, I.H.; 1991; *Quality assurance as a tool to reduce losses in animal feed production*; Advance Feed Technology; Nr. 6; p. 6-23.

Blair, M.; 1996; *Liquid or dry? A question of practicalities*; Feed Milling International; Nr. Oct.; p. 13-14.

References

Campbell, G.L. and M.R. Bedford; 1992; *Enzyme applications for monogastric feeds: a review*; Canadian journal of animal science; Ottawa; Vol. 72; Nr. 3 (Sept); p. 449-466.

Coolen, R.; 1998; Analist TNO-ILOB Zodiac; Wageningen, The Netherlands; Personal communication.

Coops, M.G.; 1997; *Bulk-blenden, Mini-symposium Cebeco Ingenieursbureau*; de Molenaar; Vol. 100; p. 2-4.

Cowan, W.D.; 1993; *Application system for the application and control of enzyme products in animal feed*; Journal of Science in Food Agriculture; Vol. 63; p. 103-113.

Eijsermans, G.W.M.; 1997; Export assistant Wijnveen (Feed Milling, Powder Processing); Ede, The Netherlands; Personal communication.

Ferraza, J, W. Bartell and R. Schick; 1992; *Spray nozzle drop size: How to evaluate measurement techniques and interpret data and reporting procedures*; Spraying Systems Co.; Wheaton, United States; 11 p.

Fodge D., A. Smith, C. Redman, H. Yu Hsiao and B. Treidl; 1997; *Post-pelleting application of heat-labile products explored*; Feedstuffs; Vol. 69; Nr. 40 29. Sept.; p. 18-26

Gadient, M., E. Schai and G. Weber; 1994; *Use of liquid carbohydrases and other additives for animals*; Proceedings 3th Kahl Symposium; Hamburg, Germany.

Gengler, L.; 1996; *Tarwe voeren zelden vetpot, Alleen bij eigen teelt is graan in het rantsoen lonend*; Varkenshouderij; Vol. 81; Nr. 15; p. 4-VA – 7-VA.

Gill, C; 1994; *Post-processing micro liquids*; Feed International; Nr. May; p. 4-6.

Günther, C. and R. Beudekker; 1997; *Die Verwendung von Enzymen in Post-Pelleting-Applikatoren*; Die Mühle + Mischfuttertechnik; Vol. 134; Nr. 18; p. 543-546.

Haaker, G; 1996; *PAON cursus mengen en agglomereren: Karakterisering van korrelvormige materialen*; Putten, The Netherlands; 27 p.

Harker, A.J.; 1995; *Application of liquid enzymes in poultry feeds*; Feed Compounder; Nr. June/July.

Hamers, S.M.W.O.M.; 1996; *Dinissen powdertechnology, lezing 23 mei 1996, doseren, vermengen, toevoegen van vaste en vloeibare componenten*; Dinissen; Sevenum, The Netherlands; 30 p.

Heeres, H.L. and J.L. Vahl; 1997; *Verwerking van toevoegings- en diergeneesmiddelen in de praktijk, GMP-code mengvoederbereiding, module 2*; p. 16-22

Heidenreich, E. and R. Löwe; 1994; *Salmonellen-Dekontamination von Futtermitteln durch Expandieren und Doppelpressen*; Die Mühle + Mischfuttertechnik; Vol. 131; Nr. 51/52; p. 701-709.

Heidenreich, E.; 1995; *Mixing technology with the view to liquid addition and cross contamination*; Victam '95, Symposium: From Feed to Food; Utrecht, The Netherlands; 6 p.

Heidenreich, E.; 1998; *Zugabe von Futterzusatzstoffen und die Gefahr von Verschleppungen*; Die Mühle + Mischfuttertechnik; Vol. 135; Nr. 10; p. 297-300.

Heijnen, G.; 1998a; *Trends in der Mischfutter-Technologie: Mischereinsatz direkt vor der Verladung*; Die Mühle + Mischfuttertechnik; Vol. 135; Nr. 4; p. 117.

Heijnen, G.; 1998b; *Technological and nutritional aspects of safe food production: Additive addition at the last moment*; Victam '98, Symposium: Safe Feed Safe Food; Utrecht, The Netherlands; 8 p.

Huber, T and M. Gadient; 1998; F. Hoffman La Roche Ltd.; Basel, Swiss; Personal Communication.

König, H.G.; 1995; *Salmonellen-Dekontamination mit dem Expander*; Die Mühle + Mischfuttertechnik; Vol. 132; Nr. 19; p. 312-316.

Kühn, I.; 1998; *New Findings on the Impact of Probiotics in Animal Nutrition*; Feed Magazine/Kraftfutter; Nr 4; p. 140-144.

Liebert, F., V.J. Nissinen and M. Peisker; 1993; *Futterenzyme in thermisch behandeltem Geflügelfutter*; Die Mühle und Mischfuttertechnik; Vol. 130; Nr 37; p. 453-454.

Limper, J.; 1998; *The Role of Amino Acids in Animal Nutrition*; Feed Magazine/Kraftfutter; Nr. 4; p. 134-136.

Lucht, H.A.; 1997; *Zusatz flüssiger Mikro-Komponenten im Mischfutterwerk*; Die Mühle + Mischfuttertechnik; Vol. 134; Nr. 4; p. 107-110.

McCoy, R.A., K.C. Behnke, J.D. Hancock and R.R. McEllhiney; 1994; *Effect of Mixing Uniformity on Broiler chick Performance*; Poultry Science; Vol. 73; p. 443-451.

Makkink, C; 1998; *Antibioticum-vrij voer, emotie of noodzaak?-Provimi symposium*; de Molenaar; Vol. 101; Nr. 14; p. 9, 11.

Nijskens, F.; 1993; *Effecten van proces-technologische behandelingen op de stabiliteit en verdeling van additieven en mogelijkheden voor verbetering, deel B: experimenteel onderzoek*; Department Animal Nutrition; Wageningen, The Netherlands; 39 p.

Nijland, R.; 1998; *De rem op groeivoer*; de Volkskrant: appendix Wetenschap; 17 oktober 1998; p. W1.

Nissinen, V.J.; 1994; *Enzymes & Processing*; International Milling Flour & Feed; Nr. May; p. 32, 33

Ouwerkerk, K.; 1997; Research & Development Wijnveen (Feed Milling, Powder Processing); Ede, The Netherlands; Personal communication.

Perry, F.G.; 1997; *Practical consideration of the usage of enzymes in pig and poultry nutrition!*; personal communication.

Peisker, M.; 1993; *Sprühsystem für flüssige Mikrokomponenten*; Kraftfutter; Nr 11; p. 538-540.

Peisker, M.; 1995; *Dosierung und Verteilung flüssiger Mikrokomponenten auf Mischfuttermittel*; Die Mühle + Mischfuttertechnik; Vol. 132; Nr. 19; p. 335-339.

Peisker, M.; 1998; *Innovative Strength of the Feed Additive Branch*; Feed Magazine/Kraftfutter; Nr 4; p. 116-125.

Putnam M. and A. Taylor; 1997; *Vitamins in feeds - the critical factors*; Feed tech; Vol. 1; Nr. 1; Document-number 108107; p. 39-41, 43.

Rensink, E; 1998; *Schone alternatieven voor antibiotica*; de Molenaar; Vol. 101; Nr. 9; p. 42-44.

Røsjorde, K: 1992; *Mixing Seminar*; Halvor Forberg A.S.; Larvik, Norway;

Robohm, K.F.; 1998; *Entwicklungtendenzen im mischfutterverarbeitenden Gewerbe*; Die Mühle + Mischfuttertechnik; Vol. 135; Nr. 7; p. 218-220.

References

Schneider and Betz; 1991; *Tests for the animal nutrition laboratory*; BASF; Ludwigshafen, Germany; 60 p.

Schneider, F.W.; 1998; *Das niederländische GMP-Regelwerk: Maßnahmen zur Verminderung und Vermeidung der Verschleppung von kritischen Produkten in der Futtermittelproduktion*; Die Mühle + Mischfuttertechnik; Vol. 135; Nr. 22; p. 740-742.

Schwarz, G; 1998a; *Liquid Feed Additives, an Alternative in Modern Animal Nutrition? (Part I)*; Feed Magazine/Kraftfutter; Nr 10; p. 438-443.

Schwarz, G; 1998a; *Liquid Feed Additives, an Alternative in Modern Animal Nutrition? (Part 2)*; Feed Magazine/Kraftfutter; Nr 11; p. 506-511.

Steen, M; 1998; *Increasing the Flexibility of Outloading*; Feed Magazine/Kraftfutter; Nr 2; p. 55-59.

Van Aken, A.M.; 1996; *PAON cursus mengen en agglomereren: Classificatie en selectie criteria voor actieve mengers*; Putten, The Netherlands; 38 p.

Van den Boogaard, A.E.J.M.; 1998; *Antibiotica: geneesmiddel of veevoederadditief?*; de Molenaar; Vol. 101; Nr. 13; p. 26-30.

Van der Ploeg, H.; 1994; *Lyxasan Symposium (4) – Gist-brocades*; de Molenaar; Vol. 97; Nr. 1; p. 11-16.

Van der Poel, A.F.B.; 1996; *Verwerking van vloeibare toevoegingen (< 1%)*; Department Animal Nutrition; Agricultural University; Wageningen, The Netherlands; 5 p.; Not published.

Van der Poel, A.F.B.; 1997; *Mengvoedertechnologie*; Department Animal Nutrition, Agricultural University; Wageningen, The Netherlands; 51 p.

Van der Poel, A.F.B. and G.M.A. Engelen; 1998; *Technological and nutritional aspects of safe food production: Post-pelleting applications (PPA) of liquid additives*; Victam '98, Symposium: Safe Feed Safe Food; Utrecht, The Netherlands; 9 p.

Van der Steege, P.; 1998; *Bulk-blending, the solution?*; Feed Magazine/Kraftfutter; Nr 5; p. 188-192.

Van Dijck P.W.M. and C. Geerse; 1993; *Feed enzymes. In: Enzymes, tools for success*. Gist-brocades bsd; Delft, The Netherlands.

Van Laarhoven, H.; 1998; *Vijftien jaar inventief vloeistoffen doseren*; de Molenaar; Vol. 101; Nr. 11; p. 28-31.

Van Leeuwen E.; 1998; Director Van Leeuwen Kwaliteitsvoeders; Puiflijk, The Netherlands; Personal communication.

Van Vliet, H.; 1998; *Gevaren van voederadditieven*; de Molenaar; Vol. 101; Nr. 16; p. 16, 17.

Von Gerlach, M.; 1992; *Verbesserung der Arbeitsgenauigkeit bei der Mischfutterherstellung durch flüssige Zusatzstoffe*; Die Mühle + Mischfuttertechnik; Vol. 129; Nr. 20; p. 277-282.

Wagner, F; 1998; *Die VICTAM aus der Sicht der Tierernärung*; Die Mühle + Mischfuttertechnik; Vol. 135; Nr. 14; p. 461, 462.

Whitehead, C.C.; 1993; *Vitamin supplementation of cereal diets for poultry*; Animal Feed Science and Technology; Vol. 45; Nr. 1; p. 81-95.

Wicker, D.L. and D.R. Poole; 1991; *How is your mixer performing?*; Feed manage; Vol. 42; Nr. 9; p. 40-44.

ANNEX A
STRESS FACTORS IN MODERN FEED PROCESSING

	Pelleting	Double Pelleting	Expander	Extruder	Anaerobic Pasteurising Conditioning (APC)	Sterilisation by Increased Retention and Temperature (SIRT)	Hydro Friction Conditioner (HFC or boa compactor)	Long term conditioner (ripener)
Temperature [°C]	70-80		130	150-170	85	95	90	
Humidity [%]	15-16			20-30			17	
Time [min]	3-5		seconds	seconds	4-5 including pressing	4-5 including pressing		20-30
Pressure [bar]			40-50	40-50				
Friction	During pressing, less than 1 minute	Higher due to higher acting time	Depending on the input of specific mechanical energy up to 20 kWh/tonne	Depending on the input of specific mechanical energy up to 100 kWh/tonne			Shearing in the outlet gap	

Reference: Heidenreich, 1995

The redox potential depends on the presence of relevant trace minerals, especially sulphates. The probability of redox reaction with double pressing is increased because of the repeated generation of active surface areas of the particles.

INDEX

ABOUT THE AUTHORS

Guus Mathias Antonius Engelen (Guus) was born on 15 September 1975 in Tegelen, Limburg, The Netherlands. He spent his youth at his parents' farm with pigs and arable land in Arcen.

In 1993 he started his study of Agricultural Engineering at the Wageningen Agricultural University and did extra classes in economics and animal nutrition. In 1998 he finished his first graduation thesis on mechanical ventilation in pig houses for the Farm Technology Group of the Wageningen Agricultural University. This thesis gained the KIvI price for the best thesis course-year 1997-1998 (Koninklijk Instituut voor Ingenieurs department mechanical and ship engineering). Also in 1998 he went to South Africa to do his practical period. In October he finished a second graduation thesis, which he started in October 1997 on the technology of liquid additives in post pelleting applications, including practical experiments in a paddle mixer at the Wageningen Feed Processing Centre for the Animal Nutrition Group (Wageningen Agricultural University). In November 1998 he graduated as an Agricultural Engineer.

Antonius Franciscus Bernardus van der Poel (Thomas) was born on 19 August 1953 in Geldrop, The Netherlands.

He has been at the Wageningen Agricultural University since 1984 where he gained his PhD in 1990 on the subject: Effects of processing on bean (Phaseolus vulgaris L.) protein quality. As an associate professor of animal feed science and technology, he teaches and lectures on feedstuffs, feed additives, concentrates, animal feed technology and least cost formulation. His research includes work on thermal processing, antinutritional factors and dry/liquid addition of additives. He is the managing director of the Wageningen Feed Processing Centre, where he is responsible for the acquisition/co-ordination of research projects, technical services and reports.